Responding to
Incidents Involving
PERSONS WITH SPECIAL NEEDS

*A Manual for
First Responders*

BARBARA J. MORVAY

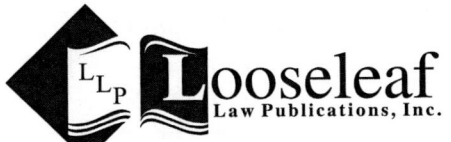

43-08 162nd Street
Flushing, NY 11358
www.LooseleafLaw.com
800-647-5547

This publication is not intended to replace nor be a substitute for any official procedural material issued by your agency of employment nor other official source. Looseleaf Law Publications, Inc., the author and any associated advisors have made all possible efforts to ensure the accuracy and thoroughness of the information provided herein but accept no liability whatsoever for injury, legal action or other adverse results following the application or adoption of the information contained in this book.

©2019 by Looseleaf Law Publications, Inc. All rights reserved. No part of this book may be reproduced, stored in a retrieval system, or transcribed, in any form or by any means, electronic, mechanical, photocopying, recording, or otherwise, without the prior written permission of the Copyright owner. For such permission, contact Looseleaf Law Publications, Inc., 43-08 162nd Street, Flushing, NY 11358, (800) 647-5547, www.LooseleafLaw.com.

Library of Congress Cataloging-in-Publication Data
Names: Morvay, Barbara J., author.
Title: Responding to incidents involving persons with special needs : a manual for first responders / by Barbara J. Morvay.
Description: Flushing, NY : Looseleaf Law Publications, Inc., 2019. | Includes bibliographical references and index.
Identifiers: LCCN 2019002539 (print) | LCCN 2019003933 (ebook) | ISBN 9781608852116 (ebook) | ISBN 9781608852109 | ISBN 9781608852116 (digital)
Subjects: LCSH: People with mental disabilities. | First responders. | Emergencies.
Classification: LCC HV3004 (ebook) | LCC HV3004 .M64 2019 (print) | DDC 362.4/0481--dc23
LC record available at https://lccn.loc.gov/2019002539

Cover by: *Looseleaf Law Publications, Inc.*

Table of Contents

About the Author i

Preface ii

Dedications ii

Chapter One 1
    A Call to Action 1
        §1.1. Setting the Scene 1
        §1.2. Victimization by the Numbers 3
        §1.3. Deinstitutionalization 4
        §1.4. The Impact of Mental Illness on Law Enforcement Response 5
    KEY POINTS 9

Chapter Two 11
    Law & Analysis 11
        §2.1. Defining "Special Needs" 11
        §2.2. The Americans with Disabilities Act of 1990 (ADA) 12
        §2.3. Disabilities as Determined by the Social Security Administration 16
        §2.4. A Timeline of Supplementary Legislation 18
    KEY POINTS 24

Chapter Three 27
    Terminology & Ideology 27
        §3.1. Introduction: Euphemisms and Political Correctness 27
        §3.2. Autism Spectrum Disorder (ASD) 29
        §3.3. Deaf-Blindness 31
        §3.4. Deafness 31
        §3.5. Emotional Disturbance 36
        §3.6. Hearing Impairment 36
        §3.7. Intellectual Disability 37
        §3.8. Multiple Disability 37
        §3.9. Orthopedic Impairment 37
        §3.10. Other Health Impaired 38
        §3.11. Specific Learning Disabilities 38
            (a) *Auditory Processing Disorders* 39
            (b) *Aphasia* 39

        (c) *Dyscalculia* 39
        (d) *Dysgraphia* 40
        (e) *Dyslexia* 40
        (f) *Dyspraxia* 40
        (g) *Sensory Processing Disorder* 40
        (h) *Visual Processing Disorder* 40
  §3.12.   Dementia 41
  §3.13.   Alzheimer's Disease 44
  §3.14.   Mental Illness 48
  KEY POINTS 52

Chapter Four 57
  WHAT'S IN A NAME? 57
  §4.1.   A Brief History 57
           The Greatest Showman 60
           Pejorative Terms 62
  §4.2.   Disability Etiquette 65
  §4.3.   Helpful Tips 66
  §4.4.   Disability Terminology 67
  KEY POINTS 69

Chapter Five 71
  RESPONSE & ASSESSMENT – PART I 71
  §5.1.   Introduction 71
  §5.2.   Some Alarming Statistics 73
  §5.3.   Addiction and Drug-Related Issues 76
  §5.4.   Individuals with Autism Spectrum Disorder 78
  §5.5.   Alzheimer's and Dementia 95
  §5.6.   Blind and Visually Impaired 105
  §5.7.   Deafness and Hearing Impairment 111
  KEY POINTS 117

Chapter Six 121
  RESPONSE & ASSESSMENT – PART II 121
  §6.1.   Mental Illness 121
  §6.2.   Intellectual Disability 129
  §6.3.   Multiple Disabilities 142
  §6.4.   Orthopedic Impairment 148
  §6.5.   Other Health Impaired 155
  §6.6.   Specific Learning Disabilities 155
  §6.7.   Traumatic Brain Injury 158
  §6.8.   Breathing Issues 160
  KEY POINTS 163

Chapter Seven 167
    ADMISSIONS AND CONFESSIONS 167
        §7.1.   Introduction 167
        §7.2.   The *Miranda* Rights 168
        §7.3.   The Formula 170
        §7.4.   Volunteered Statements 171
        §7.5.   Custody in General 171
        §7.6.   Interrogation in General 173
        §7.7.   *Miranda* and On-the-Scene Questioning 178
        §7.8.   *Miranda's* "Public Safety" Exception 178
        §7.9.   Asserting the Right to Silence or the Right to Counsel 179
            (a) *The right to remain silent* 179
            (b) *The right to counsel* 180
        §7.10. Waiver of Rights 183
            (a) *Voluntariness — a two-step analysis* 184
            (b) *A free and unconstrained choice; inducements to confess* 185
            (c) *Lying to a suspect* 185
            (d) *Juveniles and intellectually impaired individuals* ... 188
            YOUTH RIGHTS FORM 188
            (e) *Intoxicated suspects* 192
            (f) *Persons with dementia* 192
            (g) *Persons with intellectual disabilities* 195
            The Affirmative Dilemma 201
        §7.11. Outside Influences 204
            The Deity Dilemma 205
    KEY POINTS 207

Chapter Eight 211
    OBTAINING CONSENT TO SEARCH 211
        §8.1.   Introduction 211
        §8.2.   The Right to Refuse Consent 213
        §8.3.   Determining Whether the Consent Was Voluntary or Coerced 214
        §8.4.   Express or Implied Consent 217
        §8.5.   Common Authority 217
        §8.6.   Co-occupants 218
        §8.7.   The Scope of the Consent 219
        §8.8.   Obtaining Consent in Special Cases 220
            (a) *Obtaining consent from a minor* 220
            (b) *Obtaining consent from the elderly* 220

  (c) *Obtaining consent from the injured, intoxicated, drugged or those in ill health* 222
  (d) *Obtaining consent from persons with diminished capacity* 222
 KEY POINTS 229

Chapter Nine 231
REPORT WRITING IN SPECIAL CASES 231
 §9.1. Introduction 231
 §9.2. Proper Documentation 232
 §9.3. Maintaining a Proper Frame of Reference 232
 §9.4. Ensure Proper Tone 234
 §9.5. Field Notes 237
 §9.6. Body-Worn Cameras 238
 §9.7. Report Writing Checklist 240
 §9.8. Be Sure to Include All Relevant and Necessary Facts 241
 §9.9. Avoid Legal, Medical and Other Improper Conclusions 243
 §9.10. Avoid Shorthand Expressions 244
 §9.11. Avoid Inappropriate Inferences 245
 §9.12. Remain Objective 246
 §9.13. The Use of Appropriate Words 248
 §9.14. Keep It Short and Simple 255
 KEY POINTS 257

Chapter Ten 259
WHERE DO WE GO FROM HERE? 259
 §10.1. No Encounter Is the Same 259
 §10.2. The Legislative Initiative 259
 §10.3. Public Safety Policy 261
 §10.4. Who Are the People in Your Neighborhood? 263
 §10.5. An Ongoing Analysis 266
 §10.6. An Ongoing Effort 266

Glossary 269

References & Resources 285

Index 299

About the Author

Barbara Morvay has been an educator for over 37 years. She began her career as a teacher and speech therapist serving disabled children. She later became an administrator of special education, a principal and retired as the superintendent of a county school district for children with special needs. Ms. Morvay has taught as an adjunct professor at a college and university in New Jersey.

Ms. Morvay was appointed by a New Jersey governor to the Stockton University Board of Trustees, and was also appointed by a subsequent governor to the New Jersey Council for Medical Research and Treatment of Autism. She has authored two books on Autism: *My Brother is Different* and *My Sister is Different*. Ms. Morvay has dedicated her career to helping the disabled community. This book deals with essential issues of how first responders can appropriately and safely respond to people with special needs.

Preface

Determining whether an individual has a disability is a difficult task. Add to that difficulty is the fact that law enforcement officers out in the field many times need to make split-second decisions in tense, rapidly evolving situations. Keep in mind that an individual with a disability may act out or behave differently than others at the scene. Always be alert to those differences.

The suggested methods, techniques and processes in this book may be used at any time to help a law enforcement officer, firefighter, paramedic, EMT and other first responders determine rudimentary and basic functional capabilities of an individual with special needs. While they seem to be very simple, remember that the measurement of intellectual capacity and emotional intelligence is not an exact science. The methods are meant as a simple, quick guide to assist the officer in dealing with an individual with special needs. It is not a measurement device but a simple quick reference to provide helpful tips on what to do or not do when responding to incidents involving persons with special needs.

Dedications

Dedicated to all the first responders who made the ultimate sacrifice in making our world a safer place.

AND

Dedicated to those individuals who work tirelessly with people who have special needs; who strive to keep them safe and help them reach their full potential.

FOR

My children and grandchildren, love you forever and always.

Chapter One
A Call to Action

§1.1. Setting the Scene

You are dispatched to a scene with gunshots fired. Upon arrival, you observe three men fleeing from the scene. You and your partner are able to apprehend two of the individuals. Another squad car has arrived on the scene and the officers are providing support to secure the scene, and the situation starts calming down. At that point, you observe another individual huddled on the ground. The individual is exhibiting unusual behavior. He is rocking back and forth and appears to be singing to himself. As you approach to determine his condition, the rocking behavior increases. You ask, "Are you hurt?" The individual does not respond to your question. You ask again, "Are you hurt?" As you get closer, the individual's behavior intensifies; he begins to hit himself in the chest with his hand. What do you do? How do you handle the situation? The best advice in this circumstance is to step back and observe. Does the intensity of the behavior lessen? If it does, you established a comfortable space for the individual and you may deal with him without harm.

Advising you to step back may go against your instinct to approach and intervene. Do not try to stop the behavior, this may escalate the individual's self-stimulating behavior. For certain individuals who are disabled or who have special needs, behavior such as this may be a self-soothing and calming mechanism. At this point, responding officers should limit physical contact, because some disabled individuals cannot cope with touching. This individual has already demonstrated increased agitation when you got too close. Speak to him in a calm voice, don't talk loud or yell. At this point the crime scene is under control. Explain that you are there to help.

Understanding that a person with special needs may not be able to respond appropriately is essential. In an intense law enforcement incident or in an encounter with a firefighter, such an individual may not understand what is happening. They may not be able to effectively communicate and may appear to be more of a threat because of their noncompliance, which may be "non-willful." As "suspects," such individuals may not understand commands or instructions. They may be overwhelmed, confused or fearful. They may nod their head in a yes or no manner; however, this may not indicate a consistent yes or no response. They may have difficulty describing facts or details and will often demonstrate confusion. The individual could have a cognitive or verbal impairment. Here, it is important to remember that noncompliance is not the basis for violence.

Cognitive or verbal impairment is not visible. Persons with autism, communication disorders, or sensory or processing disorders are more difficult to deal with from a law enforcement perspective, particularly due to a lack of criminal culpability. In short, they have no *mens rea*. An officer faced with this situation in the field needs to first secure the individual for his safety and the safety of the officer and others nearby. In this regard, the initial encounter with the person is the most critical time period. Here, the ability to de-escalate the encounter is of utmost importance, and additional training to assist officers in dealing with the disabled in this regard is essential. If the officer is able to effectively respond to and communicate with the individual, the situation may be safely de-escalated.

While dealing with disabled and special needs children is not easy, dealing with adults with special needs or who are disabled is much more challenging. Knowing how to recognize someone with special needs or disabilities is important. Knowing how to effectively and safely respond to the situation is critical. How is this done? The answer is training. This book provides useful strategies, interventions and methods to assist law enforcement officials and other first responders in exercising safe control of a situation and how to bring it to a successful conclusion. The most essential element is always safety—the safety of the special needs individual as well as the official managing the situation.

Throughout this book, real life events will be used for instructional purposes. Practical guidelines are best explained when

A Call to Action

applied to actual events. Each year the number of encounters law enforcement professionals, first responders, firefighters, and EMTs have with the special needs population continues to increase. For the purposes of this book anyone and everyone who has a special need or a disability is included. Why? The answer is simple, the statistics support the need for training.

§1.2. Victimization by the Numbers

The following statistics from a recent report of the government Bureau of Statistics speak for themselves.[1]

- *The rate of violent victimization against persons with disabilities* (29.5 victimizations per 1,000 persons age 12 or older) *was 2.5 times higher than the rate for persons without disabilities* (11.8 per 1,000) in 2015.

- Each year from 2009 to 2015, the rate of violent victimization against persons *with* disabilities was at least twice the age-adjusted rate for persons *without* disabilities.

- One in five disabled violent crime victims believed they were targeted because of their disability.

- During 2011–15, persons with cognitive disabilities had the highest victimization rate among the disability types measured for total violent crime (57.9 per 1,000 persons age 12 or older with disabilities), serious violent crime (22.3 per 1,000), and simple assault (35.6 per 1,000).

- Persons with hearing disabilities (15.7 per 1,000) had the lowest rate of total violent victimization among the disability types examined during this period.[2]

---

[1] https://www.bjs.gov/content/pub/pdf/capd0915st_sum.pdf. For the full report (Crime Against Persons with Disabilities, 2009–2015—Statistical Tables, NCJ 250632), refer to www.bjs.gov.

[2] https://www.bjs.gov/content/pub/pdf/capd0915st_sum.pdf. For the full report (Crime Against Persons with Disabilities, 2009–2015—Statistical Tables, NCJ 250632), refer to www.bjs.gov.

§1.3. Deinstitutionalization

One of the most significant movements that changed the course of the severely mentally ill and severely disabled was the government's "deinstitutionalization" policy, which began in the mid-1950s. Deinstitutionalization was the name given to the policy through which the severely mentally ill, the severely cognitively impaired, and persons with multiple severe disabilities were moved out of large state institutions. As a result, many of the state facilities that served a real need closed. There was a belief that in doing this, patients could be served by their communities and that significant money could be saved in the process. Public psychiatric hospitals in every state began to close. There were significantly less alternative facilities, community resources, and available placements for these populations.

Some experts believe that the deinstitutionalization policy changed the health care system. According to the Treatment Advocacy Center Report of December 2015: "the system that once delivered psychiatric care to mentally ill patients has been dismantled over the last half-century."[3] Psychiatric facilities that once provided housing, medication, support and treatment for the severely mentally ill began to close.

Deinstitutionalization gave more rights to many of the higher functioning individuals who learned to cope with life's challenges and live outside the institution. However, many of those released were ill-equipped to function outside of the institution without the support and treatment of the facility. Even though the facilities provided services to the severely mentally ill, "an additional 10 to 15 percent were diagnosed with organic brain diseases—epilepsy, strokes, Alzheimer's disease, and brain damage secondary to trauma. The remaining individuals residing in public psychiatric hospitals had conditions such as mental retardation with psychosis, autism and other psychiatric disorders of childhood, along with alcoholism and drug addiction with concurrent brain damage."[4]

---

[3] htttp://www.treatmentadvocacycenter.org/storage/documents/overlooked-in-the-underground/The Role of Mental Illness in Fatal Law Enforcement Encounters, p.1.

[4] https://www.pbs.org/wgbh/pages/frontline/shows/asylums/special/excerpt.html. *Deinstitutionalization: A Psychiatric Titanic.*

A Call to Action

People were placed in the community who had no idea how to function independently without sufficient support and treatment.

The true impact of the deinstitutionalization policy is seen by law enforcement officials every day on the streets of America. Some experts believe that the policy contributed to the huge mental health crisis in this country. Hence, the *Psychiatric Titanic*.

> Deinstitutionalization further exacerbated the situation because once the public psychiatric beds had been closed, they were not available for people who later became mentally ill, and this situation continues up to the present.[5]
>
> For a substantial minority, however, deinstitutionalization has been a Psychiatric Titanic. Their lives are virtually devoid of "dignity" or "integrity of body, mind, and spirit." "Self-determination" often means merely that the person has a choice of soup kitchens. The "least restrictive setting" frequently turns out to be a cardboard box, a jail cell, or a terror-filled existence plagued by both real and imaginary enemies.[6]

§1.4. The Impact of Mental Illness on Law Enforcement Response

Given the prevalence of mental illness in police shootings, reducing encounters between on-duty law enforcement and individuals with the most severe psychiatric diseases may represent the single most immediate, practical strategy for reducing fatal police shootings in the United States.[7]

> *"The transfer of responsibility for persons with mental illness from mental health professionals to law enforcement officers is both illogical and unfair and harms both the patients and the officers."*
> Treatment Advocacy Center
> See Note 10

---

[5] *Id.*
[6] *Id.*
[7] htttp://www.treatmentadvocacycenter.org/storage/documents/overlooked-in-the-underground/The Role of Mental Illness in Fatal Law Enforcement Encounters, p.1.

Many people with mental illness and disabilities may be found on the streets across the United States and some are a part of the homeless population. Unfortunately, included in the homeless population are many U.S. Veterans who have served this country. David A. Iverson, MD, calls these vets "The Army of Lost Souls," in his article in the *Journal of Ethics of the American Medical Association*.[8] The article points out some difficult truths. "Homelessness and untreated health problems among U.S. veterans cause much public unease and, frankly, some embarrassment. Why can't society take proper care of those who risked their lives in our name?"[9]

The following statistics in the article, *The Role of Mental Illness in Fatal Law Enforcement Encounters*,[10] supports and demonstrates the significance of how mental illness effects the criminal justice system:

- **1 in 4 of all fatal police encounters involve the mentally ill.**

- **1 in 5 of all jail and prison inmates are mentally ill.**

- **1 in 10 of all law enforcement responses involve the mentally ill.**[11]

Similarly, the National Institute of Mental Health reports that *"America's jails and prisons have become our new mental hospitals."*[12] The report emphasizes that *people with mental illnesses are three times more likely to be in the criminal justice system than in hospitals*. This reflects a 90% decrease in the number of state hospital beds over the past half century.[13]

The National Institute of Mental Health is now providing some funding that will examine the effectiveness of specialized training for

---

[8] David A. Iverson, MD, Marilyn Cornell, MS, MSW and Paul Smits, MSW, The "Army of Lost Souls," http://journalofethics.ama-assn.org/2009/01/msoc1-0901.html.

[9] David A. Iverson, MD, Marilyn Cornell, MS, MSW and Paul Smits, MSW, The "Army of Lost Souls," http://journalofethics.ama-assn.org/2009/01/msoc1-0901.html.

[10] htttp://www.treatmentadvocaycenter.org/storage/documents/overlooked-in-the-under ground/The Role of Mental Illness in Fatal Law Enforcement Encounters, p.1.

[11] htttp://www.treatmentadvocaycenter.org/storage/documents/overlooked-in-the-under ground/The Role of Mental Illness in Fatal Law Enforcement Encounters, p.1.

[12] http://nimh.gov/health/statistics/index (emphasis added).

[13] http://nimh.gov/health/statistics/index (emphasis added).

law enforcement professionals. Their goal is to help respond to this population in an appropriate manner. In the meantime, law enforcement officials, firefighters, EMTs, TSAs, and first responders are dealing with intense situations that are significantly more challenging and life threatening than in the past. Many times, persons with special needs and disabilities are involved, which may present a more difficult situation for everyone.

A confrontation with a person with disabilities can escalate quickly. Knowing how to contain the situation, de-escalate it whenever possible, and maintain safety is essential. It is all too common to hear of an encounter that went wrong. If someone uses a cell phone to capture the encounter it may go viral. The media will play these negative images over and over. There are far too many incidents with special needs individuals that have "gone wrong." One need only watch the news or read a newspaper to be aware of the encounters. However, no one takes a video of a situation that is handled well and safely, that's boring. People do not video boring. The media does not put boring video on the news, it's not sensationalized. There are no YouTube videos of successful and safe encounters with people who have special needs. Officers, first responders, and firefighters in the field need assistance in handling these challenging situations now. The men and women who are tasked with safeguarding the public must be provided with sufficient resources and the necessary tools for an appropriate response.

"Police have become the default responders to mental health calls," wrote David Perry and Lawrence Carter-Long, who analyzed police incidents with the mentally ill from 2013 to 2015.[14]

Presently, only a few states are requiring legislation for the establishment of specific training in special needs and disabilities for the law enforcement community, first responders, and firefighters. More states are now recognizing the need to adopt practices and require instruction and training in this important area for the professionals who put their lives on the line every day. This book is

---

[14] https://www.nbcnew.com.../half-people-killed-police-suffer-mental-disability-report... Mar 15, 2016.

a resource tool to meet those specific requirements, hence the name of this chapter, *A Call to Action*. Effective response and safety is achieved only through education and training.

This book will provide an essential tool for instruction and training on the topics outlined above in a simple format. Learning the strategies and techniques and utilizing the helpful tips and guidelines presented will assist the law enforcement community, fire and rescue personnel, and other first responders who are the tasked with the critical job of safeguarding the public. In an emergency situation, time is of the essence, and officials need to quickly identify and ensure the safety and cooperation of persons who are disabled or who have special needs. Real life examples of compelling situations will be included, which will provide foundations for learning how to handle these challenging encounters.

A Call to Action

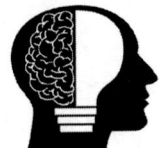

KEY POINTS

- Over a billion people about 15% of the world's population have some form of disability.[15]
- Between 110 million and 190 million adults have significant difficulties in functioning.
- Rates of disability are increasing due to population aging and increases in chronic health conditions among other causes.
- People with disabilities have less access to health care services and therefore experience unmet health care needs.[16]

"Over a billion people are estimated to live with some form of disability. This corresponds to about 15% of the world's population. Between 110 million (2.2%) and 190 million (3.8%) people 15 years and older have significant difficulties in functioning. Furthermore, the rates of disability are increasing in part due to aging populations and an increase in chronic health conditions."[17]

"Disability is extremely diverse. While some health conditions associated with disability result in poor health and extensive health care needs others do not. However all people with disabilities have the same general health care needs as everyone else and therefore need access to mainstream health care services. Article 25 of the UN Convention on the Rights of Persons with Disabilities (CRPD) reinforces the right of persons with disabilities to attain the highest standard of health care without discrimination."[18]

---

[15] World Health Organization, Key Facts, January 16, 2018, http://who.int./news-room/fact-sheets/detail/disability-and-health.
[16] *Id.*
[17] *Id.*
[18] World Health Organization, Key Facts, January 16, 2018, http://who.int./news-room/fact-sheets/detail/disability-and-health.

KEY POINTS (Continued)

In sum we all know someone with a disability. Most people are able to identify people with obvious disabilities, these are visible disabilities such as a person in a wheelchair or a person using a walker. We notice someone using a white cane as an indication of a blind or partially sighted individual. The difficulty lies in the identification of a person with an invisible disability or persons who require special needs that are not classified as disabled.

Throughout this book we will refer to both types of individuals that require special needs.

- *"HOW"* the person became disabled or has special needs is not relevant for our purposes.

- The *"WHO"* is relevant; it is anyone requiring special assistance.

- The immediate concern is the *"WHAT"* — What actions must be taken to ensure the safety of all and the de-escalation of the incident. The response, and the follow-through is essential during the incident as well as the critical follow-up documentation of the incident.

- The documentation is the *"WHY"* — it explains the specifics of why the decisions were made and justifies the actions taken.

Often, details are left out of the incident or operations report that describe the incident, the behavior of the person, and what specifically led the official to make the determination that the individual had special needs. All of these elements are important in the decision-making process. A detailed report can effectively explain what happened, why it happened and protect the officials involved. The effective documentation of the incident is critical in ensuring an accurate description of the events that took place. Situations can quickly spiral out of control; and since many incidents with "special needs" individuals can and do hit the media, effective detailed documentation can save a career.

Chapter Two
LAW & ANALYSIS

§2.1. Defining "Special Needs"

First, we need to establish a working definition for "special needs." A person with "special needs" is anyone who has an impaired ability to carry out the activities of daily living independently. This is very broad definition. Yet within this definition, one may find the various definitions for a multitude of disabling conditions. Anyone, at any time in their lifetime, may require special needs. How is this possible? If you give it some thought, the statement makes sense. A baby must have total care at birth, as the child grows they become more independent.

For example, the following circumstances or events in someone's life may dictate the requirement for special needs: a postsurgical patient; someone recovering from an illness, an accident, a significant trauma; even the elderly. Any of those circumstances may require special needs, but in such cases, there is a distinct difference—the particular circumstance is time specific. The person's period of special needs has a beginning and an end; it is not lifelong. On the other hand, people with a disability have special needs for their lifetime. This is a significant difference.

A disability can occur *prenatally, perinatally* or *postnatally. In utero,* or *prenatal,* a fetus may not develop properly due to a variety of factors, too numerous to mention here, which could lead to a lifelong disability. During the birth process, *perinatal,* something could go terribly wrong, leading to a lifelong disability. After birth, or *postnatal,* a traumatic event may occur to a baby or child leading to a lifelong disability. This is a heartbreaking event that can shatter families. Children may be born perfectly fine and develop a disability later in life due to an unfortunate circumstance. Disabilities can happen to anyone, and they can occur from a variety of factors, including hereditary factors, congenital impairments, a disease, an inflammatory condition, a degenerative condition, as well as from traumatic or developmental events.

There are common factors that define the word disability, yet there are many definitions and they are as clear as mud. How does the federal government define a disability? The federal government defines disability in multiple places, and not always in the same manner, which adds to the confusion.

The federal guidelines and definitions may be found in the following laws:

- The Americans with Disabilities Act of 1990 (ADA)[1]
- The Social Security Administration Disability Guidelines
- Section 504 of the 1973 Rehabilitation Act[2]
- The Education of All Handicapped Children Act[3]
- The "No Child Left Behind" Act of 2001 (NCLB)[4]
- The Individuals With Disabilities Education Act (IDEA)[5]
- The Every Student Succeeds Act (ESSA)[6]
- The Civil Rights of Institutionalized Persons Act (CRIPA)[7]

We will examine the diverse definitions of disabilities by the federal government below.

§2.2. The Americans with Disabilities Act of 1990 (ADA)[8]

The purpose of the ADA was to provide a clear and comprehensive national mandate for the elimination of discrimination against individuals with disabilities. According to the Act:

---

[1] Act of July 26, 1990, P.L. 101-336, 104 *Stat.* 327, popularly referred to as the Americans with Disabilities Act of 1990, which appears generally as 42 U.S.C. §§ 12101 *et seq.*
[2] Codified at 29 U.S.C. § 794.
[3] P.L. 94-142; rev. P.L.115-196, *app.* 7-7-18; codified in Title 20 *U.S.C.* §1415. Note that the *Education of All Handicapped Children Act* was later amended and renamed the IDEA. See Pub. L. 101-476, §901(a), 104 Stat. 1141.
[4] 115 Stat. 1425; codified in Title 20 U.S.C. § 6842
[5] Codified at 20 U.S.C. § 1400 *et seq.*
[6] Pub. L. No. 114-95, 129 Stat. 1802, 2171 (2015).
[7] Codified at 42 U.S.C. § 1997 *et seq.*
[8] 42 U.S.C. §§ 12101 *et seq.*

(1) physical or mental disabilities in no way diminish a person's right to fully participate in all aspects of society, yet many people with physical or mental disabilities have been precluded from doing so because of discrimination; others who have a record of a disability or are regarded as having a disability also have been subjected to discrimination;

(2) historically, society has tended to isolate and segregate individuals with disabilities, and, despite some improvements, such forms of discrimination against individuals with disabilities continue to be a serious and pervasive social problem;

(3) discrimination against individuals with disabilities persists in such critical areas as employment, housing, public accommodations, education, transportation, communication, recreation, institutionalization, health services, voting, and access to public services; and

(4) unlike individuals who have experienced discrimination on the basis of race, color, sex, national origin, religion, or age, individuals who have experienced discrimination on the basis of disability have often had no legal recourse to redress such discrimination.

42 *U.S.C.* §12102. Definition of Disability. As used in this Act:

(1) *Disability.* The term "disability" means, with respect to an individual—

(A) a physical or mental impairment that substantially limits one or more major life activities of such individual;

(B) a record of such an impairment; or

(C) being regarded as having such an impairment (as described in paragraph (3)).

(2) *Major life activities*:

(A) **In general**. For purposes of paragraph (1), major life activities include, but are not limited to, caring for oneself, performing manual tasks, seeing, hearing, eating, sleeping, walking, standing, lifting, bending, speaking, breathing, learning, reading, concentrating, thinking, communicating, and working.

(B) **Major bodily functions**. For purposes of paragraph (1), a major life activity also includes the operation of a major bodily function, including but not limited to, functions of the immune system, normal cell growth, digestive, bowel, bladder, neurological, brain, respiratory, circulatory, endocrine, and reproductive functions.

(3) *Regarded as having such an impairment*. For purposes of paragraph (1)(c):

(A) An individual meets the requirement of "being regarded as having such an impairment" if the individual establishes that he or she has been subjected to an action prohibited under this Act because of an actual or perceived physical or mental impairment whether or not the impairment limits or is perceived to limit a major life activity.

(B) Paragraph (1)(c) shall not apply to impairments that are transitory and minor. A transitory impairment is an impairment with an actual or expected duration of 6 months or less.

(4) *Rules of construction regarding the definition of disability*. The definition of "disability" in paragraph (1) shall be construed in accordance with the following:

(A) The definition of disability in this Act shall be construed in favor of broad coverage of individuals under this Act, to the maximum extent permitted by the terms of this Act.

Law & Analysis 15

(B) The term "substantially limits" shall be interpreted consistently with the findings and purposes of the ADA Amendments Act of 2008.

(C) An impairment that substantially limits one major life activity need not limit other major life activities to be considered a disability.

(D) An impairment that is episodic or in remission is a disability if it would substantially limit a major life activity when active.

(E) (i) The determination of whether an impairment substantially limits a major life activity shall be made without regard to the ameliorative effects of mitigating measures such as —

    (I) medication, medical supplies, equipment, or appliances, low-vision devices (which do not include ordinary eyeglasses or contact lenses), prosthetics including limbs and devices, hearing aids and cochlear implants or other implantable hearing devices, mobility devices, or oxygen therapy equipment and supplies;

    (II) use of assistive technology;

    (III) reasonable accommodations or auxiliary aids or services; or

    (IV) learned behavioral or adaptive neurological modifications.

(ii) The ameliorative effects of the mitigating measures of ordinary eyeglasses or contact lenses shall be considered in determining whether an impairment substantially limits a major life activity.

(iii) As used in this subparagraph —

(I) the term "ordinary eyeglasses or contact lenses" means lenses that are intended to fully correct visual acuity or eliminate refractive error; and

(II) the term "low-vision devices" means devices that magnify, enhance, or otherwise augment a visual image.

42 U.S.C. § 12103. Additional definitions. As used in this Act:

(1) *Auxiliary aids and services.* The term "auxiliary aids and services" includes—

(A) qualified interpreters or other effective methods of making aurally delivered materials available to individuals with hearing impairments;

(B) qualified readers, taped texts, or other effective methods of making visually delivered materials available to individuals with visual impairments;

(C) acquisition or modification of equipment or devices; and

(D) other similar services and actions.

* * * *

§2.3. Disabilities as Determined by the Social Security Administration

The Social Security Administration has specific guidelines for the determination of a "disability." It has established program descriptions and listings of Impairments for Adults (Part A) and a listing for Children (Part B). This information is taken directly from the Social Security Administration website at http://ssa.gov/disability and may be found in the succeeding paragraphs.

Law & Analysis

The Social Security Administration (SSA) manages two programs that provide benefits based on disability: The Social Security Disability Insurance Program (Title II of the Social Security Act (Act)) and the Supplemental Security Income (SSI) program (Title XVI of the Act).

Title II provides for payment of disability benefits to disabled individuals who are "insured" under the Act by virtue of their contributions to the Social Security trust fund through the Social Security tax on their earnings, as well as to certain disabled dependents of insured individuals. Title XVI provides SSI payments to disabled individuals (including children under age 18) who have limited income and resources.

The Act and SSA's implementing regulations prescribe rules for deciding if an individual is "disabled." SSA's criteria for deciding disability may differ from the criteria applied in other government and private disability programs.

The SSA Definition of Disability

For all individuals applying for disability benefits under Title II, and for adults applying under Title XVI, the definition of disability is the same:

> The inability to engage in any substantial gainful activity (SGA) by reason of any medically determinable physical or mental impairment(s) which can be expected to result in death or which has lasted or can be expected to last for a continuous period of not less than 12 months.

Disability in Children. Under Title XVI:

> A child under age 18 will be considered disabled if he or she has a medically determinable physical or mental impairment or combination of impairments that causes marked and severe functional limitations, and that can be expected to cause death or that has lasted or can be expected to last for a continuous period of not less than 12 months.

The SSA's List of Adult Impairments [9]

- Musculoskeletal System
- Special Senses and Speech
- Respiratory Disorders
- Cardiovascular System
- Digestive System
- Genitourinary Disorders
- Hematological Disorders
- Skin Disorders
- Endocrine Disorders
- Neurological Disorders
- Mental Disorders.
- Congenital Disorders that Affect Multiple Body Systems

The SSA's list of Childhood Impairments [10]

- All the above adult listings plus the following additions:
- Low Birth Weight and Failure to Thrive
- Cancer (Malignant Neoplastic Diseases)
- Immune System Disorders.

§2.4. A Timeline of Supplementary Legislation

1972

The Supplemental Security Income Program (SSI) was established in 1972. It is a program that pays benefits to qualified disabled adults and children who have limited income and resources. It was signed into law on October 30, 1972, and went into effect in January of 1974. The specifics may be found above.

---

[9] For a comprehensive listing, refer to:
https://www.ssa.gov/disability/professionals/bluebook/AdultListings.htm
[10] For a comprehensive listing, refer to:
https://ssa.gov/disability/professionals/bluebook/ChildhoodListings

1973

Section 504 of the 1973 Rehabilitation Act was the first disability civil rights law to be enacted in the United States. It prohibits discrimination against people with disabilities in programs that receive federal financial assistance and set the stage for enactment of the Americans with Disabilities Act.

1975

The Education for All Handicapped Children Act[11] was enacted by the United States Congress in 1975. This law had a transformative impact on millions of children with disabilities in each and every state in the country. The legislation required that public schools who received federal funds provide children with physical and mental disabilities a free and appropriate public education in the least restrictive environment. "Before this law, 'more than 1 million children with disabilities had been excluded entirely from the educational system.' The law also supported children with disabilities who had only limited access to the education system and were denied an appropriate education."[12] School districts were required to evaluate and test the children and create an Individualized Educational Plan with parental input.

Accordingly, this Act significantly changed education in the United States, disabled children were finally getting the opportunity to go to school. These issues of improved access became guiding principles for further advances in educating children with disabilities over the last quarter of the 20th century.[13]

---

[11] *P.L.* 94-142; codified in Title 20 *U.S.C.* §1415.

[12] Thirty-five Years of Progress in Educating Children with Disabilities Through IDEA. Archived: https://www2.ed.gov/about/offices/list/osers/idea35/history/index_pg10.html.

[13] *Id.*

1980

The Civil Rights of Institutionalized Persons Act (CRIPA) of 1980 has, as its stated purpose, the protection of the rights of people in state or local correctional facilities, nursing homes, mental health facilities and institutions for people with intellectual and developmental disabilities. Congress enacted this Act in 1980 to enable the Department of Justice (DOJ) to protect the rights of people residing in state institutions. The law authorizes the Attorney General to initiate or intervene in lawsuits in federal court to vindicate the rights of people in state-run or locally operated jails and prisons, juvenile correctional facilities, public nursing homes, mental health facilities, and institutions for people with intellectual disabilities. (Codified at 42 U.S.C. §1997 et. seq.)

1990

The Individuals with Disabilities Education Act (IDEA). This Act was originally known as the Education of Handicapped Children Act, which was passed in 1975. In 1990, amendments to the law were passed which changed the name to IDEA. In 1997 and again in 2004, additional amendments were passed to ensure equal access to education. The specifics of the law make available a free appropriate public education to eligible children with disabilities throughout the nation and ensures special education and related services to those children. The IDEA governs how states and public agencies provide early intervention, special education, and related services to more than 6.5 million eligible infants, toddlers, children, and youth with disabilities.

Infants and toddlers (birth through age two) with disabilities and their families receive early intervention services under IDEA Part C. Children and youth ages three through 21 receive special education and related services under IDEA Part B.[14]

---

[14] https://sites.ed.gov/IDEA/about-idea/

1990

The Americans with Disabilities Act of 1990 has, as its stated purpose, to provide a clear and comprehensive national mandate for the elimination of discrimination against individuals with disabilities. A more detailed explanation of the ADA may be found in the beginning of this chapter.

2001

The No Child Left Behind Act of 2001 (NCLBA)[15] was designed to close the achievement gap with accountability, flexibility, and choice, so that no child is literally left behind. Through the NCLBA, Congress reauthorized the Elementary and Secondary Education Act; it included Title I provisions applying to disadvantaged students; and it supported standards-based education reform based on the premise that setting high standards and establishing measurable goals could improve individual outcomes in education.

The Act required states to develop assessments in basic skills. To receive federal school funding, states had to give these assessments to all students at select grade levels. The act did not assert a national achievement standard; rather, each state developed its own standards. In this regard, the NCLBA expanded the federal role in public education through further emphasis on annual testing, annual academic progress, report cards, and teacher qualifications, as well as significant changes in funding.

Although the bill passed in the Congress with bipartisan support, it turned out to be such an unpopular law that, by 2015, the overwhelming criticism of the law caused Congress to strip away the national features of it. In fact, one school administrator referred to the law as the "No Child Left Unpunished Act."[16] The NCLBA was replaced by the Every Student Succeeds Act,[17] and was turned over to the states to administer.

---

[15] 115 Stat. 1425; codified in Title 20 U.S.C. § 6842.
[16] Superintendent, Atlantic County Special Services School District, Mays Landing, NJ.
[17] 114 *P.L.* 95; 129 Stat. 1802, 2171 (2015).

2004

Reauthorization of IDEA. Under the IDEA, a plaintiff must file his or her request for an impartial due process hearing within two years of the date he or she became aware of the actions upon which her or his claims are based. The 2004 reauthorization of IDEA, which became effective July 1, 2005, amended the IDEA to include 20 U.S.C. §1415(f)(3)(C), which provides:

> (C) *Timeline for requesting hearing.* A parent or agency shall request an impartial due process hearing within 2 years of the date the parent or agency knew or should have known about the alleged action that forms the basis of the complaint, or, if the State has an explicit time limitation for requesting such a hearing under this subchapter, in such time as the State law allows.[18]

2015

In December, 2015, Congress amended the *Individuals with Disabilities Education Act* (IDEA) through P.L. 114-95, renaming it the *"Every Student Succeeds Act."*[19] In the law, Congress states:

> Disability is a natural part of the human experience and in no way diminishes the right of individuals to participate in or contribute to society. Improving educational results for children with disabilities is an essential element of our national policy of ensuring equality of opportunity, full participation, independent living, and economic self-sufficiency for individuals with disabilities.[20]

The Individuals with Disabilities Act, IDEA, establishes specific special education categories. In order to qualify for special education

---

[18] 20 U.S.C. §1415(f)(3)(C). Prior to the 2004 reauthorization, IDEA did not have a statute of limitations. *See Pub. L. No.* 108-446, 118 Stat. 2647.
[19] *Pub. L. No.* 114-95, 129 Stat. 1802, 2171 (2015).
[20] *See* 20 U.S.C. § 1400(c)(1); *see also* https://sites.ed.gov/IDEA/about-idea/.

Law & Analysis

services a student must fall into one of the categories listed below and it must adversely affect their educational performance. If a child does not qualify for services under IDEA, they may qualify for modifications under Section 504 of the American Disabilities Act of 1973. In this regard, the goal of special education law is for a child to achieve success despite their disability.

- Autism
- Deaf-blindness
- Deafness
- Emotional Disturbance
- Hearing Impairment
- Intellectual Disability
- Multiple Disabilities
- Orthopedic Impairment
- Other Health Impairment
- Specific Learning Disability
- Speech or Language Impairment
- Traumatic Brain Injury
- Visual Impairment, Including Blindness

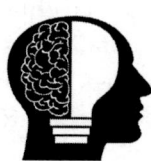

KEY POINTS

A person with a **disability** has a physical or mental impairment that substantially limits one or more major life activities.

A person with **special needs** is anyone who has an impaired ability to carry out the activities of daily living independently.

Those circumstances or events in a person's life that may generate a *temporary* requirement for special needs include: postsurgical therapy; recovering from an illness, an accident, or any significant trauma.

A disability can occur *prenatal, perinatal* or *postnatal.*

Physical or mental disabilities in no way diminish a person's right to fully participate in all aspects of society, yet many people with physical or mental disabilities have been precluded from doing so because of discrimination.

Discrimination against individuals with disabilities persists in such critical areas as employment, housing, public accommodations, education, transportation, communication, recreation, institutionalization, health services, voting, and access to public services.

The goal of the **Special Education Law (IDEA)** is for a child to achieve success despite their disability.

Law & Analysis

KEY POINTS (Continued)

Impairment of major life activities as determined by the **American with Disabilities Act** include, but are not limited to:

- Breathing
- Seeing, hearing
- Speaking
- Eating, sleeping
- Walking
- Caring for oneself
- Performing manual tasks
- Standing, lifting, bending
- Thinking, concentrating, reading, learning
- Communicating
- Working

The Federal Laws on Disabilities include:

- The Americans with Disabilities Act of 1990
- The Social Security Administration Disability Guidelines
- Section 504 of the 1973 Rehabilitation Act
- The Education of All Handicapped Children Act
- The "No Child Left Behind" Act of 2001 (NCLB)
- The Individuals With Disabilities Education Act (IDEA)
- The Every Student Succeeds Act (ESSA)
- The Civil Rights of Institutionalized Persons Act (CRIPA)

KEY POINTS (Continued)

The Individuals with Disabilities Act, IDEA, have identified specific special education categories:

- Autism
- Deaf-blindness
- Deafness
- Emotional Disturbance
- Hearing Impairment
- Intellectual Disability
- Multiple Disabilities
- Orthopedic Impairment
- Other Health Impairment
- Specific Learning Disability
- Speech or Language Impairment
- Traumatic Brain Injury
- Visual Impairment, Including Blindness

Chapter Three
TERMINOLOGY & IDEOLOGY

§3.1. Introduction: Euphemisms and Political Correctness

In this chapter, we will examine the meanings of the terms associated with various disabilities. At the outset, it is important to note that there are other factors that may fall into the category of special needs that are not addressed specifically in the law and are not included in Chapter Two, but have relevance, and will be included here. Whenever one deals with the terms describing special needs and disabilities, the challenge is the delicate balance between truth versus the euphemism. There will always be the need to modify an unpleasant or harsh description with a euphemistic phrase. Sometimes the term's modification is such that the original meaning is lost. The very definition of euphemism explains its actual purpose: "the substitution of an agreeable or inoffensive expression for one that may offend or suggest something unpleasant."[1] The terms used to describe people and children with disabilities frequently change and are modified according to society's sensibilities at the time. Euphemisms are used every day to soften difficult language. Their use has become commonplace.

"Euphemisms are unpleasant truths wearing diplomatic cologne."[2]

Here are some examples of euphemisms in everyday language:

Euphemism	Actual Meaning
Correctional facility	Jail
Passed away	Died
Senior citizen	Old person

---

[1] https://www.merriam-webster.com/dictionary/euphemism.
[2] Quentin Crisp: https://www.quotes.net/quote/5003.

Euphemism	Actual Meaning
Downsizing	Fired
Pre-Owned Vehicle	Used car
In the family way	Pregnant
Misspoke	Lied
Temporary negative cash flow	Broke
Adult beverages	Booze
Fell off the back of the truck	Stolen
Sanitation engineer	Trashman (or Janitor)
Administrative assistant	Secretary
Culinary Assembly Engineer	Fast food worker

People have also begun to use euphemistic terms to describe people with disabilities and special needs to the point of total confusion. Sometimes the words are so obtuse that no one knows what the words mean. Instead of helping to describe a person it just leads to more uncertainty.

The current "politically correct" terms used to describe the disabled and special needs population can and will change tomorrow. Recognizing that some of the terms that are found in the existing federal laws may not be acceptable to some is understandable. Some of the terms included in this book may change with time, however, these are the words that are presently in use. One must recognize that the terminology and definitions in this chapter are presently used in the federal law. They may be considered by some to be outdated or offensive, yet, until the federal laws modify or update the terminology those terms must be used.

The definitions of disabilities set forth below may be found at the government's Individuals with Disabilities Education Act's website.[3]

Many of the categories found below and the conditions described within may continue throughout a child's life and may still be present into adulthood. They may be diagnosed in a child but don't necessarily disappear. A child may learn how to cope with their

---

[3] https://www.sites.ed.gov/idea/regs/b/a/300.8/a.

Terminology & Ideology

diagnosis and be able to manage their issues. This is all dependent on severity. Many adults have the same issues as explained in the following section.

§3.2. Autism Spectrum Disorder (ASD)

Autism, also called Autism Spectrum Disorder (ASD), is a developmental disability significantly affecting verbal and nonverbal communication and social interaction, generally evident before age three, that adversely affects a child's educational performance.

"AUTISM IS THE FASTEST GROWING DEVELOPMENTAL DISORDER IN THE UNITED STATES."[4]

The areas that may be affected are:

- Behavior
- Communication
- Cognition
- Social Skills

Autism may also be called:

- Autistic Disorder
- Autism Spectrum Disorders (ASD)
- Pervasive Developmental Disorder (PDD)
- Pervasive Developmental Disorder Not Otherwise Specified (PDDNOS)
- Asperger's Disorder[5]

There are a multitude of behavioral characteristics an autistic person may develop. Some individuals demonstrate many of the characteristics and some may have just a few. The following list is neither inclusive nor exclusive. It is simply a guide to the most typical behaviors. There are varying degrees of autism. People with autism may be high functioning and be intellectually gifted in

---

[4] Barbara J. Morvay, *My Brother is Different: A parents' guide to help children cope with an Autistic sibling*, p. 3 (2010).

[5] *Id.*

specific areas or they may have mild, moderate or severe cognitive impairment.

A person with autism may demonstrate:

- limited social interaction
- limited eye contact
- dislike of physical contact
- a lack of awareness of their environment
- a lack of awareness of others
- a delay in speech or have limited speech
- limited understanding of spoken language
- limited use of language
- repetitive behaviors, such as finger flapping, rocking, spinning, clapping (This is self-stimulatory behavior and is also known as stimming.)
- the need for routine, may become upset if the routine is changed
- walking on tiptoe
- fascination with certain objects
- eating issues, a dislike of certain foods because of color, shape or texture [6]

A person with autism may also:

- repeatedly line up toys, objects, cards, or any object in a specific way
- have issues with clothes, shoes, etc.
- perseverate on certain objects, such as a clock, buttons, zippers, shoelaces, etc.
- have a short or long attention span
- have severe temper tantrums
- have self-injurious behaviors, such as head banging; finger, hand, or nail biting; hair pulling, etc.
- have severe atypical responses to their environment
- overreact to noise, visual stimuli, or people
- not like crowds, close spaces, elevators, escalators

---

[6] Barbara J. Morvay, *My Brother is Different: A parents' guide to help children cope with an Autistic sibling*, p. 4 (2010).

- have excessive fears of objects, places, etc.
- have cognitive impairment or cognitive limitations [7]

§3.3. Deaf-Blindness

Deaf-Blindness refers to a child with both hearing and visual disabilities. These are simultaneous hearing and visual impairments, the combination of which causes such severe communication and other developmental and educational needs that they cannot be accommodated in special education programs solely for children with deafness or children with blindness.

Each individual with deaf-blindness may have different degrees of each disability and the needs of each person are unique to them. This is one of the most severe disabilities that is lifelong and presents significant challenges to the activities of daily living. One of the most famous people who was deaf and blind was Helen Keller.

§3.4. Deafness

Deafness is a hearing impairment that is so severe that the child is impaired in processing linguistic information through hearing, with or without amplification.

Many people who are deaf and part of the deaf culture and community do not believe they are disabled. "The 'disability' label has been hotly debated in Deaf circles. Many disabled groups and disability theorists argue that, in most cases, it is not a biological limitation, but rather a social structure designed for a particular type of citizen that creates a disability. Deaf people can do everything that hearing people can do, except hear." [8] Yet numerous federal laws have determined that deafness is a disability therefore it is included as special needs in this book.

---

[7] *Id.* p.4.
[8] https://www.modeldeafcommunity.org/?smart_faq=do-deaf-people-consider-themselves-disabled.

The deaf and hard-of-hearing community may use American Sign Language for communication, which is a visual non-verbal language. The National Institute on Deafness and other Communication Disorders defines American Sign Language (ASL) "as a complete, complex language that employs signs made by moving the hands combined with facial expressions and postures of the body. It is the primary language of many North Americans who are deaf and is one of several communication options used by people who are deaf or hard-of-hearing." [9]

Another type of signed English may be used, sometimes referred to as Signed Exact English, a system of sign language used by a person who is deaf or hearing impaired. Signed English uses a sign for each word, so that the exact word of a spoken sentence is signed.

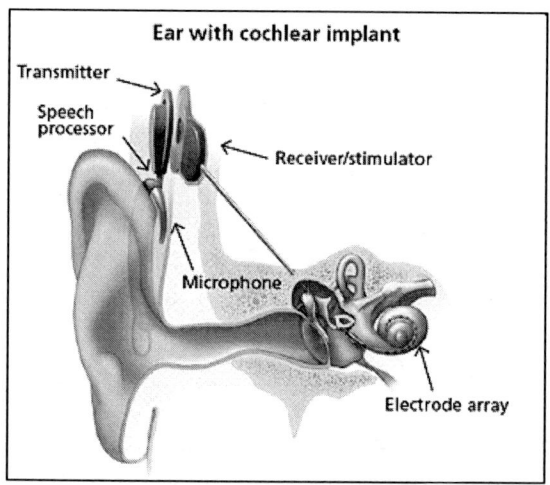
Ear with cochlear implant

Another controversial issue in the deaf culture has been the mixed reactions to the cochlear implant. There has been a great deal of emotion surrounding the issue of surgical implantation of this device. Some in the deaf community have been vehemently opposed to it and believe it could be the end of the deaf culture and American Sign Language. Regardless, with advanced technology cochlear implants are becoming more commonplace. Eventually a balance will be reached as more people who are deaf choose to get the implant.

---

[9] https://www.nidcd.nih.gov/American-Sign-Language.

What is a cochlear implant?

A cochlear implant (CI)—sometimes called a "bionic ear"—is a surgically implanted device that offers deaf people access to sound. In some cases, an implant can help a user make out spoken language. The Food and Drug Administration approved CIs for adults in 1985 and for children in 1990. As of 2016 around 96,000 people had received a cochlear implant—36,000 of them children, some as young as 12 months old.[10]

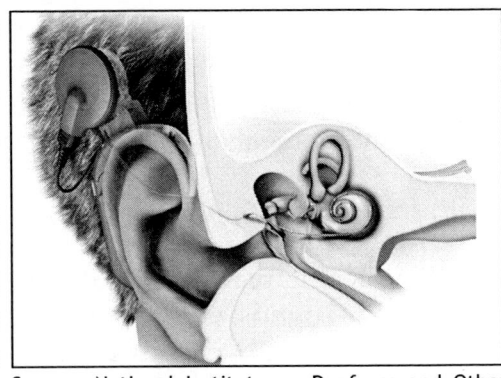

Source: National Institute on Deafness and Other Communication Disorders (NIDCD)

EXERCISE CAUTION: Law enforcement officials and other first responders should note that one portion of the device is outside the body, by the ear, and the second part is surgically attached to the skull.

https://davisfamilyhearing.com/service/cochlear-implants

This complex electronic device can help to provide a sense of sound to a person who is profoundly deaf or severely hard-of-hearing. The implant consists of an external portion that sits behind the ear and a second portion that is surgically placed under the skin *(see figure on page 33)*. An implant has the following parts:

- A microphone, which picks up sound from the environment.
- A speech processor, which selects and arranges sounds picked up by the microphone.
- A transmitter and receiver/stimulator, which receive signals from the speech processor and convert them into electric impulses.

---

[10] https://www.nidcd.nih.gov/health/cochlear-implants.

- An electrode array, which is a group of electrodes that collects the impulses from the stimulator and sends them to different regions of the auditory nerve.
- An implant does not restore normal hearing. Instead, it can give a deaf person a useful representation of sounds in the environment and help him or her to understand speech.[11]

How does a cochlear implant work?

A cochlear implant is very different from a hearing aid. Hearing aids amplify sounds, which may then be detected by damaged ears. Cochlear implants bypass damaged portions of the ear and directly stimulate the auditory nerve. Signals generated by the implant are sent by way of the auditory nerve to the brain, which recognizes the signals as sound. Hearing through a cochlear implant is different from normal hearing and takes time to learn or relearn. However, it allows many people to recognize warning signals, understand other sounds in the environment, and understand speech in person or over the telephone.[12]

Making the decision to get a cochlear implant is a very personal one. Not every person who is deaf is a candidate for the procedure. This decision is a critical one for families with newly diagnosed deaf children. The youngest recipient of a cochlear implant in the United States was 3 months old. Doctors believe that the younger the child, the better the result may be. Many factors may influence the decision for a cochlear implant such as; age, type of deafness, insurance approval, medical factors, implant center requirements, and contraindications. The field of cochlear implantation is growing as technology advances.

The deaf population may be able to read lips, make vocalizations, and speak, as well as use Sign Language. A characteristic of sign language is that it is very detailed, blunt and straightforward. Since it is a visual representation of language it is bold and describes what is seen. For example, a sign language description of someone could be: the tall, bald man with the big nose, or the old man with the big mole.

---

[11] https://www.nidcd.nih.gov/health/cochlear-implants.
[12] *Id.*

Terminology & Ideology

Many in the deaf community find the words "hearing impaired" offensive and rude. They believe that the word impaired implies that they are less than others, damaged or substandard. The deaf community believes that they are a culture that is complete with its own language and they are not less than others. The dilemma once again is that the federal laws use the terminology "hearing impairment," and that is what we are stuck with. The federal terms will be used in this book with the acknowledgment, once again, that some may find the words offensive.

Here are some things to keep in mind when interacting with a person who is deaf.

Rule Number One: Never grab a deaf person's hands.
Rule Number Two: Don't wave your hands in front of a deaf person's face.
Rule Number Three: Always keep in mind that the deaf person is keenly aware of your body language and attitude. Be respectful.

The following things are considered rude and intrusive.

Do NOT say or ask:

- You speak well for a deaf person.
- You don't look deaf.
- Can you read and write?
- I didn't know you were allowed to drive.
- Why don't you get a hearing implant?
- I'm sorry you are deaf.
- Do you really need subtitles?
- I once knew a deaf person.
- I used to have trouble with my ears.

§3.5. Emotional Disturbance

Emotional disturbance means a condition exhibiting one or more of the following characteristics over a long period of time and to a marked degree that adversely affects a child's educational performance:

(A) An inability to learn that cannot be explained by intellectual, sensory, or health factors.

(B) An inability to build or maintain satisfactory interpersonal relationships with peers and teachers.

(C) Inappropriate types of behavior or feelings under normal circumstances.

(D) A general pervasive mood of unhappiness or depression.

(E) A tendency to develop physical symptoms or fears associated with personal or school problems.

Emotional disturbance may also include schizophrenia. All of the above may also affect an adult.

It must be noted that the term "Emotional Disturbance" is most commonly referred to in education under the Special Education Federal guidelines. However, the term is also used to describe those with mental illness. Emotion disturbance may be present in varying degrees throughout a person's life.

§3.6. Hearing Impairment

When describing the term, "hearing impairment," we are referring to an impairment that is so severe that the child is impaired in processing linguistic information through hearing, with or without amplification. Please see the detailed information found above in the deaf category. Many of the same issues facing the deaf also affect the hearing impaired.

§3.7. Intellectual Disability

The term "intellectual disability" means significantly sub-average general intellectual functioning, existing concurrently with deficits in adaptive behavior and manifested during the developmental period that adversely affects a child's educational performance. The term "intellectual disability" was formerly termed "mental retardation." Intellectual disabilities are lifelong.

§3.8. Multiple Disability

The term "multiple disability" is used to describe concomitant impairments (such as intellectual disability — blindness or intellectual disability — orthopedic impairment), the combination of which causes such severe educational needs that they cannot be accommodated in special education programs solely for one of the impairments. Note that deaf-blindness is not included within the term "multiple disabilities." These disabilities are lifelong.

§3.9. Orthopedic Impairment

"Orthopedic impairment" includes impairments caused by congenital anomalies that may adversely affect a person's activities or performance. The term includes:

- impairments caused by congenital anomaly (e.g., clubfoot, absence of some member, etc.),
- impairments caused by disease (e.g., poliomyelitis, bone tuberculosis, etc.), and
- impairments from other causes (e.g., cerebral palsy, amputations, and fractures or burns that cause contractures).

The IDEA category of orthopedic impairments contains a wide variety of disorders. These can be divided into three main areas:

- neuromotor impairments
- degenerative diseases
- musculoskeletal disorders

The specific characteristics of an individual who has an orthopedic impairment will depend on the specific disease and its severity, as well as additional individual factors.

§3.10. Other Health Impaired

The term "other health impaired" refers to persons having limited strength, vitality, or alertness, including a heightened alertness to environmental stimuli, that results in limited alertness with respect to the person's surrounding environment, which is due to:

- chronic or acute health problems such as asthma
- attention deficit disorder, or attention deficit hyperactivity disorder,
- diabetes
- epilepsy
- heart conditions
- hemophilia
- lead poisoning
- leukemia
- nephritis (a kidney disorder)
- rheumatic fever
- sickle cell anemia
- Tourette syndrome

§3.11. Specific Learning Disabilities

In general, a "specific learning disability" means a disorder in one or more of the basic psychological processes involved in understanding or in using language, spoken or written, that may manifest itself in the imperfect ability to listen, think, speak, read, write, spell, or to do mathematical calculations, including conditions such as perceptual disabilities, brain injury, minimal brain dysfunction, dyslexia, and developmental aphasia.

The disorders that are not included in the specific learning disability definition include learning problems that are primarily the result of visual, hearing, or motor disabilities, of intellectual disability, of emotional disturbance, or of environmental, cultural, or economic disadvantage.

This category helps to distinguish learning disabilities from the other disability categories specified by the Individuals for Disabilities Education Act (IDEA). Specific Learning Disabilities (SLD) is by far the largest category of disability within the IDEA. Nearly half of all disabled children are labeled in the category of SLD.

Subcategories of Specific Learning Disabilities

(a) *Auditory Processing Disorders:* A common learning disability characterized by difficulty understanding spoken language. The child hears what is said but cannot process the information. Understanding and following verbal directions is difficult. A child may have difficulty following conversations and is easily distracted by noise.

(b) *Aphasia:* This condition affects speech and language. A person may have difficulty speaking or comprehending speech as well as difficulty with reading and listening. There may be problems with word retrieval, which can happen to children who have a learning disability. Many adults who have had a stroke struggle with Aphasia. They may have difficulty remembering the names of objects and also struggle with word usage and the flow of speech.

(c) *Dyscalculia:* This particular type of learning disability involves difficulty with mathematics. Children have difficulty grasping calculations, math processes and their applications. This particular type of learning disability can follow the child into adulthood.

(d) *Dysgraphia:* This learning disability involves difficulty with handwriting. Children may experience problems with holding a pencil, writing letters in words of unequal size, and spacing issues. A laptop computer can help these children and is a reasonable accommodation.

(e) *Dyslexia:* This very common learning disability involves difficulty learning to identify letters, learning to spell, read and write. Once the individual learns to write, words may be misspelled, letters and numbers may be transposed, reversed, omitted and repeated. People with dyslexia may have excellent listening skills and can be bright and articulate.

(f) *Dyspraxia:* A developmental disability that affects co-ordination. A child can have difficulty with fine and/or gross motor coordination. Issues with walking, balance and hand dexterity can occur. It may also affect speech. This condition may be lifelong.

(g) *Sensory Processing Disorder:* A neurological disorder that was originally called Sensory Integration Dysfunction whereby the brain has difficulty receiving and responding to information that comes from the one or more of the five senses. It can affect children and adults within a broad spectrum of severity. The individual may be overly sensitive to loud sounds, bright or flashing lights, touch, texture and taste. Hypersensitivity to some clothes, shoes, and food is common.

(h) *Visual Processing Disorder:* This disorder refers to the hindered ability to make sense of information seen through the eyes. The individual may have perfect vision; this is not a sight issue. It is a disorder that causes difficulty in the way the brain processes and interprets visual information. The eye may see a triangle, but the brain may interpret it as a square. Individuals may have a hard time recognizing the difference between objects, and learning letters and numbers. Learning to read could also be a challenge.

Terminology & Ideology

These explanations[13] demonstrate how a learning disability can affect a person's functional level. These issues can and do follow children for the rest of their life, they just don't fade away. It is hoped that with special education many individuals learn effective strategies and techniques to deal with their disabilities. As public service professionals, you will encounter individuals with special needs. Your challenge is to interact with these individuals in an appropriate manner, which will maintain their dignity and bring the encounter to a safe and successful conclusion.

§3.12. Dementia

No discussion of special needs would be complete without the inclusion of dementia. Law enforcement officials and other first responders are encountering more individuals with dementia than ever before. An understanding of what dementia encompasses is necessary to interact with these individuals. A diagnosis of dementia requires a comprehensive medical exam and neuropsychological evaluation. A comprehensive medical evaluation usually includes:

- Medical History and description of symptom onset
- Neurological Examination
- Laboratory Tests
- Brain Imaging — CT scan or MRI
- Mental Status Testing[14]

Dementia isn't just about simple memory mishaps — like forgetting someone's name or where you parked. A person with dementia has a hard time with at least two of the following:

- Memory
- Communication and speech

---

[13] All these categories and subcategories under specific learning disabilities may be found at the government's website: https://sites.ed.gov/idea/regs/b/a/300.8/a. The author's expanded and detailed discussion is not a part of the website.

[14] *Dementia: Is this Dementia and what does it mean?* Family Care Giver Alliance, http://www.caregiver.org/fact-sheets, June 14, 2018.

- Focus and concentration
- Reasoning and judgment
- Visual perception
    - can't see the difference in colors
    - can't detect movement
    - sees things that aren't there [15]

Dementia is diagnosed only when both memory and another cognitive function are each affected severely enough to interfere with a person's ability to carry out routine daily activities. [16]

According to the U.S. Department of Health and Human Services, there are various disorders and factors that contribute to the development of dementia. Neurodegenerative disorders result in a progressive and irreversible loss of neurons and brain functioning. Currently, there are no cures for these types of disorders.

They include:

- Alzheimer's disease
- Frontotemporal disorders
- Lewy body dementia

Other types of progressive brain disease include:

- Vascular contributions to cognitive impairment and dementia
- Mixed dementia, a combination of two or more types of dementia [17]

To make matters even more confusing, there are other medical conditions that may cause symptoms that resemble and act like

---

[15] *Alzheimer's and Dementia: What's the Difference?* reviewed by Lisa Bernstein, MD., December 26, 2016, WebMd Medical Reference, http://webmd.com.

[16] *See The Journal of the American Medical Association; see also supra,* Family Care Giver Alliance.

[17] *Types of Dementia, Basics of Alzheimer's Disease and Dementia,* U.S. Department of Health and Human Services, National Institute on Aging, http://www.nia.nih.gov, visited June 19, 2018.

dementia but are not. These conditions can be treated and the memory problems may be reversed and are as follows:

- Side effects of certain medicines
- Emotional problems, such as stress, anxiety, or depression
- Certain vitamin deficiencies
- Drinking too much alcohol
- Blood clots, tumors, or infections in the brain
- Delirium
- Head injury, such as a concussion from a fall or accident
- Thyroid, kidney, or liver problems [18]

Doctors have identified many other conditions that can cause dementia or dementia-like symptoms. These conditions include:

- Argyrophilic grain disease, a common, late-onset degenerative disease
- Creutzfeldt-Jakob disease, a rare brain disorder
- Huntington's disease, an inherited, progressive brain disease
- Chronic traumatic encephalopathy (CTE), caused by repeated traumatic brain injury
- HIV-associated dementia (HAD) [19]

Due to the similarities and the common symptoms of the various types of dementia, getting an accurate diagnosis is essential for proper treatment. People are encouraged to seek out a medical expert who specializes in dementia.

---

[18] *Id.*
[19] *Id.*

§3.13. Alzheimer's Disease

Alzheimer's Disease is the most common type of dementia. "About 60% to 80% of people who have dementia have Alzheimer's."[20] According to the United States Department of Health and Human Services, increasing age is the most important known risk factor for Alzheimer's. The number of people with the disease doubles every 5 years beyond age 65. About one-third of all people age 85 and older may have Alzheimer's disease. Late-onset Alzheimer's, the most common form of the disease, probably includes a combination of genetic, lifestyle, and environmental factors.[21]

Scientists are now learning how age-related changes in the brain may harm nerve cells. These changes may contribute to Alzheimer's. Some of the changes include atrophy (shrinking) of certain parts of the brain, inflammation, production of unstable molecules called free radicals, and a breakdown of energy production within cells. There are two types of Alzheimer's—early-onset and late-onset. Both types have a genetic component.

The Alzheimer's Association has developed a list of 10 Early Signs and Symptoms of Alzheimer's Disease. It is included in this book on page 44 with the express written permission of that group.

---

[20] See generally supra, WebMd Medical Reference.
[21] U.S. Department of Human Services, content reviewed May 22, 2017, https://www.nia.nih.gov/health/what-causes-alzheimers-disease.

Terminology & Ideology

10 Early Signs and Symptoms of Alzheimer's*

Memory loss that disrupts daily life may be a symptom of Alzheimer's or other dementia. Alzheimer's is a brain disease that causes a slow decline in memory, thinking and reasoning skills. **There are 10 warning signs and symptoms.** If you notice any of them, don't ignore them. Schedule an appointment with your doctor.

Memory loss that disrupts daily life

One of the most common signs of Alzheimer's disease, especially in the early stage, is forgetting recently learned information. Others include forgetting important dates or events, asking for the same information over and over, and increasingly needing to rely on memory aids (e.g., reminder notes or electronic devices) or family members for things they used to handle on their own.

What's a typical age-related change?
Sometimes forgetting names or appointments, but remembering them later.

Challenges in planning or solving problems

Some people may experience changes in their ability to develop and follow a plan or work with numbers. They may have trouble following a familiar recipe or keeping track of monthly bills. They may have difficulty concentrating and take much longer to do things than they did before.

What's a typical age-related change?
Making occasional errors when balancing a checkbook.

Difficulty completing familiar tasks at home, at work or at leisure

People with Alzheimer's often find it hard to complete daily tasks. Sometimes, people may have trouble driving to a familiar location, managing a budget at work or remembering the rules of a favorite game.

What's a typical age-related change?
Occasionally needing help to use the settings on a microwave or to record a television show.

---

* Reprinted with written permission from the Alzheimer's Association, https://alz.org/alzheimers-dementia/10_signs

Confusion with time or place

People with Alzheimer's can lose track of dates, seasons and the passage of time. They may have trouble understanding something if it is not happening immediately. Sometimes they may forget where they are or how they got there.

What's a typical age-related change?
Getting confused about the day of the week but figuring it out later.

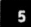
Trouble understanding visual images and spatial relationships

For some people, having vision problems is a sign of Alzheimer's. They may have difficulty reading, judging distance and determining color or contrast, which may cause problems with driving.

What's a typical age-related change?
Vision changes related to cataracts.

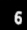
New problems with words in speaking or writing

People with Alzheimer's may have trouble following or joining a conversation. They may stop in the middle of a conversation and have no idea how to continue or they may repeat themselves. They may struggle with vocabulary, have problems finding the right word or call things by the wrong name (e.g., calling a "watch" a "hand-clock").

What's a typical age-related change?
Sometimes having trouble finding the right word.

Misplacing things and losing the ability to retrace steps

A person with Alzheimer's disease may put things in unusual places. They may lose things and be unable to go back over their steps to find them again. Sometimes, they may accuse others of stealing. This may occur more frequently over time.

What's a typical age-related change?
Misplacing things from time to time and retracing steps to find them.

Terminology & Ideology 47

Decreased or poor judgment

People with Alzheimer's may experience changes in judgment or decision-making. For example, they may use poor judgment when dealing with money, giving large amounts to telemarketers. They may pay less attention to grooming or keeping themselves clean.

What's a typical age-related change?
Making a bad decision once in a while.

Withdrawal from work or social activities

A person with Alzheimer's may start to remove themselves from hobbies, social activities, work projects or sports. They may have trouble keeping up with a favorite sports team or remembering how to complete a favorite hobby. They also may avoid being social because of the changes they have experienced.

What's a typical age-related change?
Sometimes feeling weary of work, family and social obligations.

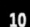

Changes in mood and personality

The mood and personalities of people with Alzheimer's can change. They can become confused, suspicious, depressed, fearful or anxious. They may be easily upset at home, at work, with friends or in places where they are out of their comfort zone

What's a typical age-related change?
Developing very specific ways of doing things and becoming irritable when a routine is disrupted.

Get checked. Early detection matters.

If you notice any of the 10 Warning Signs of Alzheimer's in yourself or someone you know, don't ignore them. Schedule an appointment with your doctor.

§3.14. Mental Illness

Mental illnesses are conditions that affect a person's thinking, feeling, mood or behavior, such as depression, anxiety, bipolar disorder, or schizophrenia. These conditions may be occasional or long-lasting (chronic) and affect someone's ability to relate to others and function each day. According to the American Psychiatric Association, "serious mental illness is a mental, behavioral or emotional disorder (excluding developmental and substance use disorders) resulting in serious functional impairment, which substantially interferes with or limits one or more major life activities."[22] Examples of serious mental illness include major depressive disorder, schizophrenia and bipolar disorder.

Although the terms are often used interchangeably, poor mental health and mental illness are not the same thing. A person can experience poor mental health and not be diagnosed with a mental illness. Likewise, a person diagnosed with a mental illness can experience periods of physical, mental, and social well-being. A person's mental health can change over time, depending on many factors. When the demands placed on a person exceed their resources and coping abilities, their mental health could be impacted. For example, if someone is working long hours, caring for an ill relative or experiencing economic hardship they may experience poor mental health.[23]

The government's Centers for Disease Control (CDC), reports that mental illnesses are among the most common health conditions in the United States. Negative attitudes and misconceptions associated with mental health and mental illness still exist. Yet the following facts demonstrate the statistics of mental illness in the United States.

---

[22] *What is Mental Illness?* American Psychiatric Association, physician reviewed by Ranna Parekh, M.D., M.P.H., November 2015, http://www.psychiatry.org/patients-families/.
[23] *Learn about Mental Health,* http://www.cdc.gov/mentalhealth/index.htm. Updated January 26, 2018.

- In 2016, there were 44.7 million adults—about 1 in 5 Americans—with a mental illness.[24]

- In 2016, there were an estimated 10.4 million adults with serious mental illness. This represents 4.2% of all U.S. adults.[25]

- Just over 20% — or 1 in 5 — children, have had a serious debilitating mental disorder.[26]

- Half of all chronic mental illness begins by age 14 and three-quarters begin by age 24.[27]

- Suicide, which is often associated with symptoms of mental illness, is the tenth leading cause of death in the U.S. and the second leading cause of death among people aged 19 to 34.[28]

These statistics speak for themselves. Consequently, the likelihood of a law enforcement officer, firefighter or EMT encountering someone with a mental illness is high. Recognizing these individuals is important, yet they are difficult to determine quickly. There is no single cause for mental illness. A number of factors can contribute to the risk of mental illness, for example:

- Early adverse life experiences, such as trauma or a history of abuse (for example, child abuse, sexual assault, witnessing violence, etc.);

---

[24] https://www.nimh.nih.gov//health/topics/index.shtml. Data presented from 2016 National Survey on Drug Use and Health (NSDUH) by the Substance Abuse and Mental Health Services Administration (SAMHSA).

[25] *Id.*

[26] Health & Education Statistics (http://www.nimh.nih.gov/health/statistics/prevalence/any-disorder-among-children.shtml) Bethesda, MD, National Institute of Mental Health, National Institutes of Health, 2016.

[27] Kessler RC, Chiu WT, Demler O, Walters EE. Prevalence, Severity, of Twelve-month DSM-IV Disorders in the National Comorbidity Survey Replication (NCS-R). Archives of general psychiatry. 2005;62(6):617-627. doi:10.1001/archpsyc.62.6.617. Substance Abuse and Mental Health Services Administration, Center for Behavioral Health Statistics and Quality (2016). Key substance use and mental health indicators in the United States: Results from the 2015 National Survey on Drug Use and Health. Rockville, MD.

[28] Rui P, Hing E, Okeyode T. National Ambulatory Medical Care Survey: 2014 State and National Summary Tables. Atlanta, GA: National Center for Health Statistics, Centers for Disease Control and Prevention, 2014.

- Experiences related to other ongoing (chronic) medical conditions, such as cancer or diabetes;
- Biological factors, such as genes or chemical imbalances in the brain;
- Use of alcohol or recreational drugs;
- Having few friends, or the wrong type of friends; and
- Having feelings of loneliness or isolation.[29]

There are more than 200 classified types of mental illness. A listing of these may be found in The Diagnostic and Statistical Manual of Mental Disorders V, (DSM-5). DSM-5 defines and classifies mental disorders and is the manual used by doctors and mental health professionals to diagnose people with mental health. The study of mental illness has evolved over the years but no one can exactly predict the behavior of others. Dealing with a person with a mental illness wielding a gun is serious and unpredictable.

The media can overly simplify news by sensationalizing events. One of the negative outcomes of this is the belief that many individuals that are mentally ill frequently engage in violent behavior. Yet studies show that the majority of individuals with mental illness are never violent. Mental illness is strongly associated with increased risk of suicide, which accounts for over half of the firearms–related fatalities in the United States.

"In the aftermath of mass shootings and other violent events, the public and policymakers look for answers to the question of how such an event could have been prevented. When the perpetrator is reported to have had a mental illness, questions arise about why he was not identified and treated before committing a major act of violence. The issue of predicting risk of future violence among people with mental illness is central to the development of policy responses to mental illness and violence. Policies intended to keep guns out of the hands of people with mental illness who are likely to be violent depend on clinicians to accurately identify *which*

---

[29] Learn about Mental Health, http://www.cdc.gov/mentalhealth/index.htm.updated January 26, 2018.

individuals are likely to be violent. However, research evidence shows that risk prediction, particularly for statistically-rare events like mass shootings, is a very inexact science." [30]

In Chapter One, an explanation of how the deinstitutionalization policy which began in the mid-1950s had a tremendous effect on the mental health crisis in the United States. Many experts have determined that this policy did not work. The direct effect has been experienced by law enforcement officials, EMTs, first responders and firefighters across the country on a daily basis.

---

[30] Mental illness and reduction of gun violence and suicide: bringing epidemiologic research to policy—Jeffrey W. Swanson, PhD, E. Elizabeth McGinty, PhD, MS, Seena Fazel, MBChB, MD, FRC Psych, and Vickie M. Mays, PhD,d, MS,PHd,e, May 2015, https://www.ncbi.nlm.nih.gov/pmc/articles/PMC4211925/

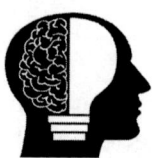

KEY POINTS

- Autism is the fastest-growing developmental disorder in the United States.

- A person with autism may demonstrate limited social interaction, limited eye contact, a dislike of physical contact, a lack of awareness of their environment and of others, along with repetitive behaviors, such as finger flapping, rocking, spinning, or clapping.

- The terms used to describe people and children with disabilities frequently change and are modified according to society's sensibilities at the time (politically correct terms or PC).

- Whenever one deals with the terms describing special needs and disabilities, the challenge is the delicate balance between truth versus the euphemism.

- Euphemisms are used every day to soften the descriptive language associated with disabilities and special needs. Their use has become commonplace, so much so, that the euphemistic terms cloud the actual meanings, leading to more confusion.

- Federal terms for the disabled are not modified quickly and may be found to be offensive by some groups.

- Many people who are deaf and part of the deaf culture and community do not believe they are disabled.

- Deaf people can do everything that hearing people can do, except hear; these individuals use American Sign Language or Signed Exact English for communication.

Terminology & Ideology

KEY POINTS (Continued)

- Law enforcement professionals, first responders, firefighters, as well as public safety officials are encountering people with special needs more frequently.
- Not all people with special needs are easily identifiable.
- Mental illnesses are among the most common health conditions in the United States.
- Negative attitudes and misconceptions associated with mental health and mental illness still exist.

The following checklist identifies the various conditions that may be found in people with disabilities and special needs. Please note that children may have the same issues as adults except they would NOT have Dementia, or Alzheimer's Disease. Sadly, they could have Alcoholism and Drug Addiction. The special needs and disability groupings have been divided into visible and invisible categories.

Visible Disabilities

___ Blind

___ Deaf with Cochlear Implant

___ Multiple Disabilities

___ Orthopedic Impairment

Invisible Disabilities

___ Autism

___ Deafness

___ Emotional Disturbance

___ Hearing Impairment

___ Intellectual Disability

___ Health Impaired

KEY POINTS (Continued)

___ Specific Learning Disabilities
◇ Subcategories:
- Auditory Processing Disorders
- Aphasia
- Dyscalculia
- Dysgraphia
- Dyslexia
- Dyspraxia
- Sensory Processing Disorder
- Visual Processing Disorder

___ Alcoholism

___ Alzheimer's Disease

___ Dementia

___ Drug Addiction

___ Mental Illness
◇ Subcategories:[31]
- Anxiety Disorders
- Bipolar Disorders
- Depression
- Eating Disorders
- Hoarding Disorders

---

[31] These subcategories are by no means all of the mental illnesses identified by The American Psychiatric Association and included in the Diagnostic and Statistical Manual of Mental Disorders (5th ed.), known as DSM-5. It is simply a list of the most common disorders that may be encountered by law enforcement officials and other first responders in the performance of their duties.

Terminology & Ideology

KEY POINTS (Continued)

- Mood Disorders
- Neurodevelopmental Disorders
- Obsessive Compulsive Disorders
- Panic Disorders
- Post Traumatic Stress Disorders
- Psychotic Disorders
- Schizophrenia
- Substance Abuse and Addiction

Chapter Four
WHAT'S IN A NAME?

§4.1. A Brief History

In a world where political correctness has become the norm, there is confusion over the terms that describe persons with special needs or disabilities. Certain words have become uncomfortable. What are the correct words? Words and actions reflect the beliefs and attitudes of a society at a specific time. In this chapter we will examine the history of how the disabled were treated and the cruel names they were called.

> *"The difference between the almost right word and the right word is really a large matter—'tis the difference between the lightning-bug and the lightning."*[1]
> *Mark Twain*
> *American Author & Humorist*

From the 1800s to the mid-1900s, many disabled people were denied education and housing. Discrimination against the disabled was everywhere—virtually universal. Some were placed in institutions and kept out of the public eye. Others were shunned; they lived on the streets. Before the advancement of medical science, no one understood the disabled. People were often fearful that they could "catch" the condition. Many disabled children and adults were kept hidden away by families. They were the subject of ridicule and disdain, and were commonly called freaks and oddities.

Even the justices of the United States Supreme Court were not above this controversy. For example, in 1927, the Court, in *Buck v. Bell*,[2] by a vote of 8 to 1, upheld the constitutionality of a Virginia law that authorized the involuntary, compulsory sexual sterilization

---

[1] Mark Twain (Samuel Clemens), Letter to George Bainton, 10/15/1888 twainquotes.com.
[2] 274 *U.S.* 200 (1927).

of "mental defectives," including the intellectually disabled, to promote the "health of the patient and the welfare of society."[3] The subject of the case, Carrie Buck, after being raised by foster parents and allegedly raped by their nephew, was declared feebleminded and promiscuous. In 1924, she was committed to the Virginia State Colony for Epileptics and Feebleminded, near Lynchburg, and was, in accordance with Virginia law, ordered to be sterilized. The Virginia legislature enacted the law as a reaction to arguments that certain social problems, including shiftlessness, poverty, and prostitution, were inherited and ultimately could be eliminated through selective sterilization. In what would become an infamous opinion, Justice Oliver Wendell Holmes, Jr., observing that Carrie Buck, her mother, and her daughter were all suspected of being feebleminded, declared: "Three generations of imbeciles are enough."[4] The curt, five-paragraph opinion was never overturned and led to a marked increase in sterilizations across the United States.[5] At the Nuremberg Trials, Nazi defendants cited *Buck v. Bell* in their own defense. As one commentator observed, "*Buck v. Bell* could represent the highest ratio of injustice per word ever signed on to by eight Supreme Court Justices, progressive and conservative alike."[6] It was not until 1974 that Virginia's General Assembly repealed the law; in 2002 the state formally apologized to its victims.[7]

In the 19th century, another disturbing phenomenon occurred when the disabled became a part of the entertainment industry and became popular "attractions" in the "freak shows" of England and the United States. During this time, "freak shows" and novelty acts caught the imagination of a larger viewing audience. People were willing to pay for the opportunity to witness human medical oddities and rare conditions. It became a booming business, as people with physical abnormalities grew into a highly profitable

---

[3] *Id.* at 205.

[4] *Id.* at 207.

[5] Two years after *Buck v. Bell* was handed down, twelve states had new sterilization laws; within four years, twenty-two more states had introduced new sterilization bills.

[6] Victoria Nourse, *Buck v. Bell: A Constitutional Tragedy from a Lost World*, 3 Pepp. L. Rev. 101-117 (2011).

[7] While *Buck v. Bell* was never overturned, the Supreme Court in *Skinner v. Oklahoma*, 316 *U.S.* 535 (1942), outlawed sterilization as a punitive measure, something the Virginia legislature was careful to repudiate in 1974.

market, particularly in England and the United States.[8] "Sideshows, or freak shows as they are sometimes referred to, contained various forms of entertainment in one evening. Every now and then, a magician would be thrown into the mix to give the crowd a brief respite from some of the more unsettling abnormalities they were witnessing. However, not all performers were 'natural' freaks born with physical deformities. Some were performance artists who had unusual talents, such as fire eating, sword swallowing or full-body tattoos."[9]

The Ringling Brothers Circus officially opened for business in 1884, and the brothers capitalized on the extreme and bizarre to earn profit. Apparently, it worked. "For many years, the most popular component of the circus was the 'Freak Show.' Though often thought of as exploitative, degrading, and cruel, most reports paint a picture of headlining 'freaks' being both accepted and well-paid by the circus staff. In many cases, the performers not only out-earned everyone in the audience, but also their own promoters. Any mistreatment generally came from the public who did not look at the performers as people."[10]

Clyde Ingalls, manager of the Ringling Brothers and Barnum & Bailey sideshow in the 1930s once said, "Aside from such unusual attractions as the famous three-legged man, and the Siamese twin combinations, freaks are what you make them. Take any peculiar looking person, whose familiarity to those around him makes for acceptance, play up that peculiarity and add a good spiel and you have a great attraction."[11] Some of the individuals who starred in the Ringling Brothers' "Freak Shows" became famous. Annie Jones, who headlined as the "Bearded Lady," had a rare genetic abnormality that caused excessive facial hair. Jack Earle, who had a genetic growth abnormality (acromegalic gigantism), was called "The World's Tallest Human," standing 8ft. 6½in. tall. There was also

---

[8] Laura Grande, *Strange and Bizarre: The History of Freak Shows,* History Magazine, October/November Issue. (9/26/2010), http://thingssaidanddone.wordpress.com/2010/9/26/strange-and-bizarre-the-history-of-freak-shows.
[9] *Id.*
[10] Erin Kelley, The Sad Stories of the Ringling Brothers' "Freak Show" Acts, May 19, 2016, updated May 4, 2018, pg. 1., http://allthatsinteresting.com/freak-show-members.
[11] *Id.* at 2.

Major Mite, who was only 2ft. 2in., and Myrtle Corbin, the four-legged girl, born with two separate pelvises, her four individual legs made her a popular oddity. Other stars of the show were "General Tom Thumb," who stood only 2 feet tall, and Fedor Jeftichew, who was called "Jo-Jo the Dog-Faced Boy." Jeftichew was born with hereditary hypertrichosis, also known as werewolf syndrome, which causes an excessive amount of hair growth over the entire body.[12] As medical science became more advanced, medical and scientific explanations of such physical abnormalities were revealed in the literature and for public consumption, and gradually, over time, these shows disappeared.

The Greatest Showman

In late 2017, the movie musical, The Greatest Showman was released, with Hugh Jackman starring as P.T. Barnum. It was loosely based on the man who created the "circus" by using "freaks" and "oddities" Hollywood style. Many of the individuals discussed in this chapter are featured in this movie, such as; The Bearded Lady, The Strong Man, The Irish Giant, The Tattooed Man, Dog Boy, The Fat Lady, The Albino Sisters, General Tom Thumb, and The Siamese Twins among others. The movie typifies how people with disabilities were used in circus and side shows and that time.

The movie emphasizes inclusion, tolerance and acceptance and is true family entertainment with all the bells and whistles of a Hollywood production. In reality, there was a lot of people that believed that P.T. Barnum and The Ringling Brothers Circus truly exploited the people with disabilities. But some people "argue that Barnum gave many of his performers a dignity they didn't, or couldn't have in their former lives, and it's fascinating to see their stories portrayed in The Greatest Showman."[13] Even though the movie is a fictionalized account, it does effectively demonstrate how people with disabilities found a home in the circus.

Another unbelievable example of the negative treatment of the disabled occurred at the Willowbrook School on Staten Island, which

---

[12] *Id.* at 3-10.
[13] https://www.bustle.com

What's in a Name?

opened in October of 1947. The governor of New York at the time, Thomas Dewey, wanted Willowbrook to be a place for "mentally and physically defective and feebleminded, who never can become members of society," who needed to be cared for with a "high degree of tenderness and affection."[14] Unfortunately the opposite happened, Willowbrook actually became a nightmare for its residents, it was a place of horrors. Willowbrook was the largest mental institution in the country. The first the American public heard of the horrors of Willowbrook was from a speech made by a promising young politician. Speaking of systemic failures in mental-health care, Robert Kennedy said "I've visited the state institutions for the mentally retarded, and I think particularly at Willowbrook, we have a situation that borders on a snake pit."[15] However, nothing was done, and Willowbrook remained open.

It wasn't until early 1972, when Geraldo Rivera, an investigative reporter for WABC-TV in New York, gained access to Willowbrook with the help of an employee. His taped report showed the deplorable conditions at the facility and may be viewed on YouTube. It must be noted that the actual footage and report is difficult to watch. Geraldo's investigative report was shown on national news and created such outrage that it helped to shut down the facility.[16] Geraldo Rivera said that the Willowbrook story was a defining moment in his life—"the residents lived in filth and squalor, some were naked and wailing in hallways smeared with feces." How do I describe the smell? He said, "filth, disease and death."[17]

It was also discovered that many of the residents were being used for human medical experiments and were injected with hepatitis without the consent of their parents. It was verified that it went on for nearly twenty years.[18] Geraldo Rivera made a significant contribution that shed light on a deplorable place and its

---

[14] Matt Reimann, *Willowbrook, the institution that shocked a nation into changing its laws, Patients needing "tenderness and affection" got the opposite*, contributing writer, (June 15, 2017), http://Timeline_Now,timeline.com.

[15] *Id.*

[16] Geraldo Rivera, http://index.geraldo.com/folio/biography.

[17] http:www.youtube.com/watch/Unforgotten:Twenty five Years After Willowbrook.

[18] Matt Reimann, *Willowbrook, the institution that shocked a nation into changing its laws, Patients needing "tenderness and affection" got the opposite*, contributing writer, (June 15, 2017) http://Timeline_Now,timeline.com.

treatment of the disabled. Fortunately, things began to change as states and the federal government enacted programs and laws to protect the rights of the disabled. A listing of these laws may be found in Chapter Two.

Pejorative Terms

The pejorative terms used to describe the disabled, which were once commonly used and accepted by society, have taken a bit longer to disappear. In the past, these offensive words were part of ordinary language.

For example:

- Afflicted
- Stricken
- Cripple
- Crip
- Gimp
- Gimpy
- Retard
- Tard
- Feebleminded
- Slow
- Mentally Defective
- Deaf and Dumb (or just Dumb)
- Lunatic
- Idiot
- Imbecile
- Mental
- Defectives

- Half Wit
- Dim Wit
- Unfit
- Dullard
- Moron
- Dull
- Spazz
- Deficient
- Sightless
- Drawler
- Shaky
- Thicko
- Mad
- Disturbed
- Goon
- Perverted
- Psycho
- Queer
- Nuts

- Nutter
- Demented
- Freak
- Loony Bin
- Crackers
- Deformed
- Brain Dead
- Screw Loose
- Mad
- Schizo
- Cretin
- Vegetable
- Nutball
- Delusional
- Fruitloop
- Eccentric
- Village idiot
- Half-baked
- Bonkers

Moreover, negative descriptive phrases associated with the disabled have been colloquialized into our everyday language.

What's in a Name?

We all have a universal understanding of the following:

- His elevator doesn't go all the way to the top.
- The lights are on but nobody's home.
- He's a few sandwiches short of a picnic.
- He's not the sharpest knife in the drawer.
- There's a village somewhere that's looking for its idiot.
- He's out of his tree.
- He's got a screw loose.
- She's not playing with a full deck.
- She's lost her marbles.
- Not quite all there, are you?
- A few bricks shy of a load.
- A few cans short of a six pack.
- He's just a half a bubble off plumb.
- The blind leading the blind.
- What are you, deaf, dumb and blind?
- He's nutty as a fruit cake.
- He's off his rocker.
- One more brain cell and he could be considered dangerous.
- A few crumbs short of a biscuit.
- A few French fries short of a happy meal.
- Did you forget your crazy pills this morning?
- He should be in the loony bin.
- That's schizo.
- He's a retard.

Clearly, these negative descriptive phrases are wholly inappropriate. As a public service professional, it is essential to recognize that certain words are still used in a context to diminish and verbally hurt someone. Various agencies for the disabled have determined that the word handicapped should no longer be utilized to describe a person with a disability. Even as we become more aware of the needs of people with disabilities, the words we use to describe disabilities have not changed in all written material. Older accepted versions of the law still exist, books with outdated terms will still be in the marketplace. Eventually some written material will be modified to reflect current accepted standards and terms. However, all literature can't be changed.

It is essential, therefore, to remember the following key points:

- People with a disability are individuals first and foremost.

- It is always wrong to be rude and call anyone a derogatory name.

- Always treat the person with respect.

- Do not assume someone who cannot speak cannot hear.

- Do not assume that someone in a wheelchair, or using a walker or cane has a cognitive impairment.

- Do not speak about the person with special needs in front of them to another individual.

One of the best examples of "not judging a book by its cover" was the acclaimed and brilliant theoretical physicist, Professor Stephen Hawking. Professor Hawking had ALS; he had extraordinary physical challenges, yet he accomplished more in his lifetime than most. What is ALS? According to the ALS Association, ALS, or amyotrophic lateral sclerosis, is a progressive neurodegenerative disease that affects nerve cells in the brain and the spinal cord. The progressive degeneration of the motor neurons in ALS eventually leads to their demise. When the motor neurons die, the ability of the brain to initiate and control muscle movement is lost. With voluntary muscle action progressively affected, people may lose the ability to speak, eat, move and breathe.

What's in a Name?

ALS is also referred to as Lou Gehrig's disease because the famous baseball great had the disease. ALS usually strikes people between the ages of 40 and 70, and it is estimated there are more than 20,000 Americans who have the disease at any given time (although this number fluctuates). For unknown reasons, military veterans are approximately twice as likely to be diagnosed with the disease as the general public. Why discuss Professor Hawking here? Because simply recognizing that someone is in a wheelchair and unable to speak does NOT mean that they do not understand. They can be alert, intelligent and aware of their surroundings. One cannot and should not make assumptions about a person who is disabled or has special needs by how they look.

§4.2. Disability Etiquette

Kenneth A. Stern wrote an excellent article entitled Disability Etiquette, wherein he explains "as we've become more sensitive to the needs of persons with disabilities, one aspect of society that has remained stubbornly behind the curve are the words we use to describe one another." [19]

It is important to recognize that long-held beliefs may still affect our response to people with special needs. "Becoming aware of our own perceptions, stereotypes and discomforts around particular disabilities is the first step towards addressing subtle biases that could possibly be projected onto individuals with disabilities," states St. Mary's County for People with Disabilities. "Our own beliefs and comfort level around disability has a major impact on how we view, interact, and provide service and programs." [20]

The following information is presented with the express written permission of Kenneth A. Stern, Esq., on June 12, 2018, as described in his article, Disability Etiquette. [21]

---

[19] Kenneth A. Stern, Disability Etiquette, http://www.cerebralpalsy.org/information/disability/etiquette/ (June 12, 2018).

[20] *Id.*

[21] Kenneth A. Stern, Disability Etiquette, http://www.cerebralpalsy.org/information/disability/etiquette/ (June 12, 2018).

§4.3. Helpful Tips

- DO NOT define someone by his or her disability.

- She is not a disabled person, she is a person with a disability (remember that one is a *person first*).

- DO NOT identify a person by the impairment or disability, unless it is relevant. Example: "The individual using the wheelchair..." is only deemed appropriate when the use of the wheelchair is relevant to the conversation.

- DO NOT use slang to label a person. He is not "crippled," "retarded," "disabled," "impaired," "spastic," or "special-ed." He is simply a person with special needs.

- Use updated terminology. Example: She is not "wheelchair-bound," "physically handicapped," "differently abled," or "physically challenged." Instead, "She uses a wheelchair," "she has a disability," or "she has a physical impairment."

- Eliminate any negative tone as it is hurtful. For example, he is not "special ed," he participates in the special education program.

- Eliminate disrespectful slang and words that imply victimization. For example, he is not a victim, unfortunate, crippled, sufferer, stricken, or an invalid. He simply has an impairment.

- A person with total hearing loss is considered a person who is without hearing.

- A person with partial hearing loss is referred to as a person with a hearing impairment.

- A person with total sight loss is not referred to as "a blind person," but as "a person who is blind."[22]

---

[22] *Id.*

What's in a Name?

- A person with a varying degree of sight—a person who can see but is not considered legally blind, for example—is a person with a vision impairment.

- A person who displays trouble speaking, uses voice prosthesis, or appears to stutter is "a person with a speech impairment."

- Also, "normal" is a word that, depending on its context, should not be used.

- It's okay to say, "It's normal to feel down once in a while." It is not acceptable to say, "John uses a walker because his legs aren't normal." A better way to express the sentiment would be, "John often uses a walker to get to and from school."

§4.4. Disability Terminology[23]

Do Use Terminology Properly

- Become aware of the proper meaning behind terms. Improper use leads to hurt feelings, offended individuals, and disrespectful use of language.

Do Respect the Person, First

- Referring to an individual by his or her impairment is no longer acceptable. Acceptable terminology accentuates the person first, then mentions his or her impairment, only if pertinent. Labeling an individual is inappropriate. Describing an individual is appropriate. Do this by placing emphasis on the person, not the person's condition. It is proper to say "person with a disability" as opposed to "disabled person." It is proper to say "person with epilepsy" versus "the epileptic." It is appropriate to state "the boy with quadriplegia" versus "the quadriplegic."

---

[23] Kenneth A. Stern, Disability Etiquette, http://www.cerebralpalsy.org/information/disability/etiquette/(June 12, 2018).

- Terms like physically challenged, differently abled, physically handicapped, and wheelchair-bound are outdated. The current trend is to limit the use of labeling terms with negative connotations. Descriptive terms without judgment are accepted. For instance, "the individual using the wheelchair."

Do Get to Know the Level of Impairment

- A person with total hearing loss is considered "a person who is without hearing," but is not considered a "deaf person." Likewise, a person with partial hearing loss is referred to as "a person with hearing impairment."

- A person with total sight loss is considered "a person who is blind," but is not considered a "blind person." A person with a varying degree of sight—a person who can see but is not considered legally blind, for example—is "a person with vision impairment." A person who displays trouble speaking, uses voice prosthesis, or appears to stutter is "a person with speech impairment." [24]

Don't Refer to the Person in a Negative Way

- Negativity is disempowering. The impairment is a condition, not a result of violence. A person should not be given a label that insinuates inappropriate treatment. For instance, do not use terms like victim, sufferer, stricken by, deformed, incapacitated, unfortunate, invalid or afflicted with. For instance, "John may have cancer," but John is never "a cancer victim."

---

[24] Kenneth A. Stern, Disability Etiquette, http://www.cerebralpalsy.org/information/disability/etiquette/(June 12, 2018).

What's in a Name?

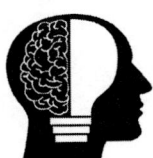

KEY POINTS

- Discrimination against the disabled and mentally ill has been around for hundreds of years.

- At one point the disabled were part of the freak shows in the United States and Europe.

- In *Buck v. Bell*, the United States Supreme Court upheld the constitutionality of a Virginia law that authorized the involuntary, compulsory sexual sterilization of "mental defectives," including the intellectually disabled, to promote the "health of the patient and the welfare of society."

- The Willowbrook Facility story that appeared on the national news shocked the nation and may have led to *The Civil Rights of Institutionalized Persons Act* (CRIPA) of 1980.

- The United States federal law CRIPA protects the rights of people in state or local correctional facilities, nursing homes, mental health facilities and institutions for people with intellectual and developmental disabilities.

- DO NOT define someone by his or her disability; remember that she is not a disabled person, she is a person with a disability (remember that one is a person first).

- Use terminology properly and refer to all persons with respect.

- Our own beliefs and comfort level around disability has a major impact on how we view, interact, and provide service and programs.

- Do not assume that someone in a wheelchair and who is unable to speak does not understand.

Chapter Five
RESPONSE & ASSESSMENT – PART I

§5.1. Introduction

In communities across the United States, law enforcement officials, fire and rescue personnel and other first responders are encountering various situations that involve disabled individuals. Once on the scene, they have to quickly assess and determine many factors in a matter of seconds. Is the person armed with a weapon? Is there a threat to themselves or others? Does someone require medical intervention? Is the person disoriented? Is the person's behavior bizarre? Officials have been trained to respond to certain crisis situations in a specific manner, but this may not work well when encountering someone with a disability.

A person with special needs may be found at the scene of a crime, may be seen wandering disoriented in a neighborhood, may be the victim of violence, may call 911, may be a bystander, may have participated in a crime, may have been involved in an accident, may have been assaulted, or may be having a medical emergency. These are just some of the possibilities that may occur. In this chapter we will identify strategies, best practices and guidelines to help officials respond to calls in a way that best supports individuals with special needs, and to ensure a positive, safe result. The goal is to avoid mistakes that could lead to negative outcomes, lawsuits and critical media attention. The challenge is to recognize that not all people with disabilities can be dealt with in the same manner. In the following pages, guidelines and suggestions for interactions with persons having specific special needs will be identified. In all cases, the severity of the disability will determine the individual's capacity to understand, speak and interact with officials.

"A person in crisis is still a person in crisis, whether they have a developmental disability or not. Everyone in crisis needs more time, more space, and less stimulation to unlock their ability to

think and cope under stress. All persons in pain, under the influence, with head injuries, with psychiatric disorders, or simply "locked up" with fear or rage can benefit from the same communication tips." [1]

As a law enforcement official, firefighter or other first responder, you will come in contact and interact with someone who has a disability. What do you do first? Determine their level of impairment. There are times when the severity of the impairment is such that it will be obvious, at other times it is not readily apparent.

CAUTION: *Your job is not to diagnose, but to observe, access and determine if a person may have special needs and modify your response accordingly.*

The recognition that an individual with special needs may require a different type of intervention is a successful beginning. The key to your interaction with a person who has special needs is situational awareness, it must be applied to every encounter.

The following guidelines may be applied to persons with other types of disabilities. The strategies are not limited to only one type of disability. People with cognitive impairment, dementia, mental illness, physical disabilities as well as the many other special needs described herein may all benefit from the principles described below. Your responsibility as an official is to protect and serve all citizens, while recognizing that interacting with the most vulnerable populations is often the most challenging.

CAUTION: *Just because a person has a disability doesn't mean that they are not dangerous. Always guard your weapons and be alert until you determine the threat assessment.*

Nonetheless, behaviors that are demonstrated by people with certain disabilities may appear as threatening or noncompliant. These actions are not defiant but simply a manifestation of their disability.

---

[1] Joel Lashley, Interventions for Patients with Challenging Behaviors Instructor, p. 4, Children's Hospital of Wisconsin, Security Services, Children's Hospital and Health Systems, Autism Spectrum Disorders: A Special Needs Subject Response for Police Officers. Form#95d2b2b5-41b9-40b5-951b-a5a3568696cc.

"If we fail to recognize what may be obvious signs of cognitive disabilities we can expect to end up in unnecessarily violent encounters. Children and adults with challenging behaviors due to neurological, psychological, and physical disabilities rely on the police to keep them safe and enforce their rights to be treated with dignity and respect and access freedoms that healthy people take for granted."[2]

§5.2. Some Alarming Statistics

According to the U.S. Department of Justice, Bureau of Justice Statistics Report of July 2017, the rate of violent victimization against persons with disabilities was 2.5 times higher than the rate for persons without disabilities.

From 2011 to 2015, persons with cognitive disabilities had the highest rates of total violent crime (57.9 per 1,000), serious violent crime (22.3 per 1,000), and simple assault (35.6 per 1,000) among the disability types measured.[3]

In 1998, The Crime Victims with Disabilities Awareness Act was passed (P.L. 105-301). It mandates that the National Crime Victimization Survey (NCVS) include the statistics on crimes against persons with disabilities and the disability characteristics of those persons. The purpose of this act was *"to increase public awareness of the plight of victims of crime with developmental disabilities, to collect data to measure the magnitude of the problem, and to develop strategies to address the safety and justice needs of victims of crime with developmental disabilities."*[4]

---

[2] Joel Lashley, *Interventions for Patients with Challenging Behaviors Instructor*, p. 4, Children's Hospital of Wisconsin, Security Services, Children's Hospital and Health Systems, Autism Spectrum Disorders: A Special Needs Subject Response for Police Officers. Form#95d2b2b5-41b9-40b5-951b-a5a3568696cc.

[3] Crime Against Persons with Disabilities, 2009–2015—Statistical Tables|July 2017, bjs.gov.

[4] *Id.* at 3.

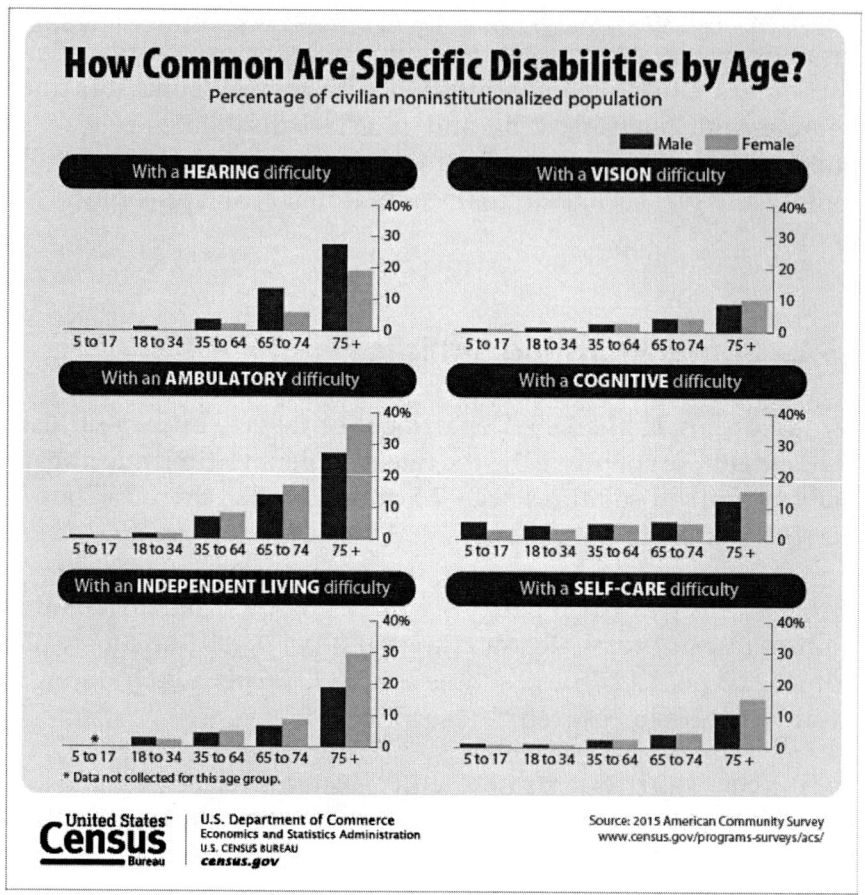

The following statistics from the Crime Against Persons with Disabilities Awareness Report, 2009–2015,[5] demonstrate how disabled individuals are more likely to be the victim of a crime than people without disabilities.

- The rate of serious violent crime (rape or sexual assault, robbery, and aggravated assault) for persons with disabilities (12.7 per 1,000) was more than three times the rate for persons without disabilities (4.0 per 1,000).

- The rate of simple assault against persons with disabilities (19.6 per 1,000) was more than twice the rate for persons without disabilities (8.7 per 1,000).

---

[5] Statistical Tables, p.4 of the July 2017 Report.

Response & Assessment - Part I

- Serious violent crime accounted for a greater percentage of violence against persons with disabilities (39%) than violence against persons without disabilities (32%).

- During 2011–15, while 49% of persons with disabilities had multiple disability types, an estimated 54% of violence against persons with disabilities occurred against those with multiple disability types.

- Sixty-five percent of rapes or sexual assaults against persons with disabilities were committed against those with multiple disability types, the highest percentage among the crime types examined.

Given those statistics, it is more likely that a law enforcement officer, firefighter or other first responder will be called to a scene where a person with a disability may be the victim of a crime rather than the perpetrator of the crime. That is not to say, however, that this is always the case. In situations where addiction and drugs are involved, crimes are committed; and it is critical to note at this juncture that this group is not included in the statistical report as having a disability.

The groups included in the report were categorized according to six limitations:

- hearing (deafness or serious difficulty hearing)

- vision (blindness or serious difficulty seeing, even when wearing glasses)

- cognitive (serious difficulty in concentrating, remembering, or making decisions because of a physical, mental, or emotional condition)

- ambulatory (difficulty walking or climbing stairs)

- self-care (a condition that causes difficulty dressing or bathing)

- independent living (physical, mental, or emotional condition that impedes doing errands alone, such as visiting a doctor or shopping).[6]

In relation to the detailed statistical data included in this section, it is advisable that when responding to a scene that involves a person with a disability, serious consideration must be given to the circumstances. An abundance of caution and attention to detail should be foremost in your mind and actions in response and assessment.

§5.3. Addiction and Drug-Related Issues

No book on *Responding to Persons with Special Needs* would be complete without an acknowledgment of the current drug epidemic in this country. The significance of the problem is such that an entire book could be written on the subject. The seriousness of the subject matter is so complex and far reaching that an adequate attempt at an explanation would be beyond the scope of this book. However, it must be mentioned herein as its impact is felt everyday by the law enforcement community.

The drug epidemic has had a serious impact on law enforcement officials, firefighters, and other first responders. Not surprisingly, because of this, the number of calls to 911 have significantly increased. When the words such as, unconscious, unresponsive, difficulty breathing, vomiting, seizures, or blue lips are used to describe someone, the odds are likely that the victim is experiencing a drug overdose. This presents risks to the first responders. Exposure to drug paraphernalia, fentanyl and its derivatives, as well as other drugs poses a threat to anyone responding to the scene. Frequently, the address is familiar to the officials because they have responded to that address in the past.

Ongoing training is needed to provide the necessary assistance in safeguarding the lives of the officials and the victims. It is recommended that law enforcement officials, firefighters, EMTs,

---

[6] *Crime Against Persons with Disabilities, 2009–2015—Statistical Tables|July 2017*, bjs.gov., page 1.

Response & Assessment - Part I

paramedics, and other first responders avoid contact with any of these substances and be trained to recognize the potential hazards. Always use personal protective equipment such as gloves, dust masks, even eye protection if you have it; these items should be carried with you since you never know when you may be called to a scene that may require these items.

> In the last several years, U.S. Law Enforcement has seen a dramatic increase in the availability of dangerous synthetic opioids. A large majority of these synthetic opioids are structural derivatives of the synthetic drug "fentanyl." Fentanyl is a synthetic opioid currently listed as a Schedule II prescription drug that mimics the effects of morphine in the human body but has the potency 50 to 100 times that of morphine. Due to the high potency and availability of fentanyl, both transnational and domestic criminal organizations are increasingly utilizing these dangerous synthetic opioids as an adulterant in heroin and other controlled substances.[7]

The DEA has put out the following warning:

> There is a significant threat to law enforcement personnel, and other first responders, who may come in contact with fentanyl and other fentanyl-related substances through routine law enforcement, emergency or life-saving activities. Since fentanyl can be ingested orally, inhaled through the nose or mouth, or absorbed through the skin or eyes, any substance suspected to contain fentanyl should be treated with extreme caution as exposure to a small amount can lead to significant health-related complications, respiratory depression, or death.[8]

---

[7] https://www.dea.gov/.../Fentanyl_BriefingGuideforFirstResponders_June2017.pdf.
[8] https://www.dea.gov/.../Fentanyl_BriefingGuideforFirstResponders_June2017.pdf.

The following examples demonstrate how officials may be exposed to dangerous drugs.

> **Milwaukee, 2018**
>
> - Three officers were treated for exposure to dangerous substances while making an arrest.
>
> - An officer was transported to the hospital after exposure to fentanyl following an arrest of a suspect where the drug was found.
>
> **Greendale**
>
> - Two officers were exposed to an unknown substance while searching a purse found in a suspected stolen vehicle. They began to experience symptoms of exposure and were administered Narcan, a drug used to combat opioid overdoses, and taken to the hospital.
>
> **Waukesha County**
>
> - A sheriff's deputy was hospitalized for drug exposure to powder during a traffic stop.

§5.4. Individuals with Autism Spectrum Disorder

The Center for Disease Control and Prevention (CDC) report of April 26, 2018, states that 1 out of 59 children (1 in 37 boys and 1 in 151 girls) have been identified as having an Autism Spectrum Disorder. Autism is 4 times more common in boys than girls.[9]

These statistics have been increasing over the past twenty years. Since autism is a lifelong disability, children with autism grow up and face significant challenges as adults. Law enforcement officials, firefighters, EMTs, paramedics, and other first responders will

---

[9] https://www.cdc.gov/ncbddd/autism/data.html.

encounter persons with autism frequently. Why? Due to their unusual behavior, people with autism may not be immediately recognizable as such, and persons encountering them may be frightened or concerned by their behavior. Frequently, someone calls 911 because they see a person who looks disoriented or unusual wandering in the community; the call was not placed because of a crime being committed. Wandering is a significant problem since the person with autism does not understand danger. This factor places the individual in situations that puts them at greater risk. It has been determined that they may be victimized more than the general population.

Autistic individuals are not all alike. There are variations in understanding, cognition, functional level, and individual response, which could be either mild, moderate or severe. Yet, they do have two important characteristics in common—their difficulty with socialization and communication. Even if the individual is non-verbal, do not assume that he cannot understand basic language. One of the most obvious signs of autism is stimming, which is self-stimulatory behaviors and unusual repetitive behaviors.

Persons with autism might demonstrate certain behaviors and characteristics. For example, they may:

- be unable to understand a dangerous situation.

- wander in a neighborhood or be drawn to bodies of water, traffic or other dangers.

- be overwhelmed by flashing lights, certain sounds, loud noises, sirens, or fire.

- be afraid of a person in uniform, or a firefighter in turnout gear.

- demonstrate curiosity and reach for objects or equipment such as a shiny badge or handcuffs or even your gun.

- react in an inappropriate manner.

- react by trying to run away or try to hide.

- not respond or understand commands such as stop or put your hands up.

- have difficulty with speech or language, or be non-verbal.

- not respond to his or her name.

- appear to be deaf.

- not make eye contact.

- act out by biting, or hit themselves or others.

- display repetitive behaviors known as stimming by rocking back and forth, hand flapping, hitting, head rolling, spinning, or other similar behaviors.

- have auditory, sensory or visual perception issues.

- have other medical issues such as a seizure disorder.

- not respond to pain in a typical way and may not be able to explain their pain.

- act very nervous, cry out or vocalize loudly, using unfamiliar sounds.

- not understand consequences, or right from wrong.

- not have a sense of modesty; therefore, undressing or inappropriate touching may be observed.

If a first responder is able to identify that a child or adult may have autism, he or she can then respond in a way that best supports the individual.

How to interact with a person who has autism.

First and foremost, assess the situation to determine if any reasonable threat exists. Remember that an autistic individual may demonstrate atypical behaviors described above. This is a characteristic of their disability not necessarily an active threat.

Response & Assessment - Part I

The most important thing to do is **LISTEN!**

If there are people around who know the person, listen to what they have to say. They may have important information about this individual, such as, he cannot speak, or the person is deaf, or he has a cognitive impairment or a seizure disorder. This information is essential to the task at hand. Their information can help de-escalate a situation.

If the autistic person has a caregiver that is present, work with them to establish a sense of safety and cooperation.

"When responding to calls involving subjects with autism, 4 out of 5 times you'll be handling a subject in crisis, who is scared and/or lost, not a criminal." [10]

Do not get too close to the person, give the person space. Getting too close may agitate the individual causing them to act out.

Determine who will be the lead professional interacting with the person, and stick with it! Ask your partner or others at the scene to step back. This is important, since the individual is already in distress and having difficulty. Having the person focus only on one person is essential.

Limit NOISE and distractions. In this regard, try to limit the amount of unnecessary chatter around the person; less talking and distractions around the person translates to faster control of the situation.

Allow space between you and the individual; getting too close may seem threatening.

Take your time with the individual. Initial contact is the point where things could go wrong. People may be watching and they all have smartphones that could video the event as it develops. Spend

---

[10] Joel Lashley, *Interventions for Patients with Challenging Behaviors Instructor*, p. 4, Children's Hospital of Wisconsin, Security Services, Children's Hospital and Health Systems, Autism Spectrum Disorders: A Special Needs Subject Response for Police Officers. Form#95d2b2b5-41b9-40b5-951b-a5a3568696cc.

the necessary time now rather than having the event portrayed in a negative way on the evening news.

Tell them your name and what you are doing. Be specific, people who are autistic do not understand things that may be obvious to other people. This process takes some time.

For example:

> *My name is John. I am here to help you.*
> Tell them who you are. Assume they do not understand what the uniform represents.

> *"I am a _____."* (fill in the blank, a police officer, sheriff's officer, a firefighter, etc.)

> Now Wait ...

> Say, *"You don't have to talk to me."*

> Repeat, *"I am here to help you."*

> *"You can shake your head or move your hand if you hear me."*

This takes the pressure off the need for verbal communication, which may be difficult. Remember the autistic individual may be in panic mode, frightened, and disoriented.

If the person responds, consistently offer praise, and say thank you.

"Thank you for letting me know you understand."

Tell them what will happen and what you will be doing before you do it. This is very important.

For example, *"I am going to walk around you to make sure you are OK."*

Response & Assessment - Part I

Recognize that even if the person appears to be hurt, they may not be able to understand. They may be confused and disoriented. They may not react to pain the same way others would.

They may have low muscle tone known as hypotonia, which can affect the brain, the central nervous system, or the muscles. Therefore, they may appear limp, which could mask serious injuries. The individual may also have a coordination disorder, which makes it difficult to access a person's physical status.

Attention to detail is of the utmost importance. Just because the individual does not seem to be aware of the injury does not mean they are not experiencing pain. When dealing with a person with autism who has an injury, the best course of action would be to call for an ambulance. At this point you would not want to transport an individual with autism in a squad car. The injuries could be more serious than they appear, and there may be underlying medical conditions that are not visible. Therefore, it is always best to get professional medical help. An abundance of caution is best in these circumstances.

It would be best for you to say, *"I see you are hurt, I am going to help you."*

Use simple sentences and speak slowly.

Do not yell. You may have to repeat your statement.

Give the person time to process and respond.

Tell the person, *"I am calling some of my friends to help."*

"They will come in an ambulance."

If possible, ask the ambulance and first responders to shut off the flashing lights and the siren as they approach the scene.

At this point, it is essential for you to stay with the autistic person. At this point, you have established a rapport with the person. You are now their caretaker. Your interactions and demeanor have provided a level of safety and the individual knows you will not hurt him. Therefore, your continued presence is necessary for a successful outcome.

Be alert to the signs of increased frustration (rocking, vocalizing, self-stimming) and try to eliminate the source if possible, thereby reducing the possibility of negative behavior.

Do not try to stop the person from their self-stimulating behavior, this may cause physical acting out and more self-injurious behavior.

Avoid using quick movements.

Limit loud noises and flashing lights if possible.

Do not touch the person unless absolutely necessary.

If you have a blanket or a towel available, offer it to the individual or place it near the person. It may provide a sense of comfort, and they may reach for it and hold on to it.

If they are sitting on the ground, bend down to their level, don't stand above them, this may be perceived as aggressive behavior.

Sometimes the autistic person may demonstrate negative behavior as an indication of a need. They may need to go to the bathroom, or they may be in pain, or cold, and hungry or afraid and may not be able to communicate that need. Try to take care of a few of their basic needs, this can change everything for the better. It would be good practice to always have a blanket or towel in your vehicle. If you do, place it near the person. It provides a sense of comfort and security as well as warmth which is important in establishing a sense of trust.

You should always try to have a bottle of water and a snack, such as crackers or pretzels or M&M's in your vehicle. Just the simple act of placing food near the person and backing away can have a positive effect. DO NOT offer food or water if the individual has any serious injuries, since this could complicate any medical procedures.

Response & Assessment - Part I

DO NOT RUSH THE PROCESS! Do not allow anyone else to rush you. This could be a career-defining moment. Right here and right now, this event could determine whether you are seen as the HERO or the VILLAIN. Give the situation the time and attention it deserves. This is not a typical encounter, it requires your utmost patience, humanity and compassion.

The following two examples of encounters gone viral effectively demonstrate two situations that went wrong. They are used here as learning tools.

Florida, July 2016; the headline read:

"Florida Cop charged with Attempted Manslaughter in Shooting of Autistic Man's Unarmed Therapist."

The Miami-Dade State Attorney's Office announced on April 17, 2017, that charges would be brought against an officer after shooting an unarmed therapist with one count of attempted manslaughter, a third-degree felony, and one count of culpable negligence, a first-degree misdemeanor after its investigation of the following incident.

The circumstances of the case began when a 23-year old man with autism, who required 24-hour supervision, wandered away from the Miami Achievement Center for the Developmentally Disabled. He left the facility holding a small, toy truck. His unarmed, behavioral therapist followed the autistic man to try and get him to return to the facility. Thereafter, a 911 caller reported a disturbed man who may or may not have a gun, who was possibly suicidal.

The man with autism sat down in the middle of the street, and played with his toy. Three police officers arrived at the scene. The therapist was talking to the autistic man, trying to coax him to return to the center. As people watched the scene unfold, a bystander began to take a video with their cell phone.

The unarmed therapist, obeys police orders and lies down on his back and raises his arms in the air. He can be heard saying to the police, *"Sir, there is no need for firearms, I'm*

> unarmed, he's an autistic guy. All he has in his hands is a toy truck, that's all – a toy truck. Please don't shoot, no need for a gun. I am a behavior therapist at a group home."[11]
>
> In the police statement regarding the incident, it was reported that three officers were at the scene, two of the officers who were 20 feet from the scene did not use their weapons. The third officer, who was about 150 feet away, fired three shots in the direction of the autistic man. It was one of those shots that struck the therapist. The officer who shot the unarmed man said that he was trying to protect him from the autistic man, who he thought was a threat, but shot the therapist by mistake. The statement issued by the Florida State Attorney's Office stated that "the third officer was not in a position to correctly assess the situation or in a position to accurately fire."[12]
>
> The video that shows the moments before the shooting went viral. It was played on the evening news, the morning news and the national news.
>
> The American Civil Liberties Union of Florida and its Miami chapter praised the decision to bring charges, saying that they hoped the North Miami police force used the shooting as a chance "to thoroughly review training and procedures" to further help respond to "situations involving individuals with mental and developmental disabilities."[13]

This incident demonstrates how quickly an encounter can escalate when law enforcement officials confront someone with a mental illness, cognitive impairment or autism. Videos of this incident and the news reports may be viewed on the following websites:

https://www.nbcnews.com/.../florida-cop-charged-manslaughter-shooting-autistic-man...

https://www.chicagotribune.com/.../ct-charges-florida-officer-shooting-20170412-story.html.

---

[11] www.chicagotribune.com/.../ct-charges-florida-officer-shooting-20170412-story.html; see also https://www.nbcnews.com/.../florida-cop-charged-manslaughter-shooting-autistic-man.

[12] www.chicagotribune.com/.../ct-charges-florida-officer-shooting-20170412-story.html.

[13] Id.

It should be noted that there was so much media attention to this event that it may have prompted officials in the State of Florida to pass an Autism Training Mandate for law enforcement officers in October of 2017.

> **Buckeye, Arizona, September 2017**
>
> While on patrol near a park, a police officer approaches a 14-year-old autistic boy. The boy is standing on the sidewalk playing with a string-manipulating the string from side to side, up and down, backwards and forwards. The officer asks the boy what he is doing; the boy responds, *"I am stimming."* The officer asks again, the boy says, *"A string."* The officer then asks, *"Do you have any ID on ya?"* The boy says *"No."* Things escalate from there. The officer tackles the boy, mistaking his mannerisms for signs of drug use, perhaps a reaction to an inhalant. The boy can be heard repeating, *"I'm okay! I'm okay!"* — a self-soothing mechanism, as the officer spins the boy around to attempt to handcuff him. All the while, the boy is saying, *"I'm okay!" I'm okay!"* When the officer forces the boy onto the ground, the boy is heard saying, *"I need help."*
>
> The boy explained to the officer he was "stimming." Stimming is a shorthand expression for self-stimulatory behavior, which can be any type of repetitive movements of body parts, objects, words, phrases or sounds. It is a common characteristic in people with autism. The officer said that the boy was displaying signs of being under the influence of an inhalant. The officer's 21-minute body cam footage shows a boy who tried to explain what he was doing. That video has gone viral. It is posted on YouTube and scenes were played on the CBS morning and evening news. As a result of the encounter with the officer, the boy sustained multiple cuts and bruises. The boy and his mother were later interviewed by a reporter.
>
> The video can be seen at:
> https://www.youtube.com/watch?v=uErofKXMwq0

> It is a difficult thing to watch. After the incident, the boy's family sent a letter to the police department asking for a few things: (1) an apology from the officer; (2) that the officer participate in an autism-related community service project; (3) more training for all the officers in the department; and (4) for the Police Department to pay the boy's medical bills, particularly for the surgery needed to repair the boy's foot. When the department failed to respond to the family, they filed a $5 million lawsuit.[14]

Firefighters, Paramedics, EMTs and Autism

When firefighters are called to a scene it is usually an emergency. Their goal in any emergency situation is to quickly get to work to insure the safety of all. In critical situations when people are in danger, autistic individuals may not act in a typical fashion. They may run and hide even if their life is at risk. The following quick facts for firefighters was developed by the Autism Speaks Organization in cooperation with W. Cannata.

Quick Facts for Firefighters, Paramedics and EMTs[15]

- Individuals with autism can't be identified by appearance.

- Some individuals with autism do not have a normal range of sensations and may not feel the cold, heat, or pain in a typical manner.

- They may fail to acknowledge pain in spite of an injury.

- They may show an unusual pain response that could include laughter, humming, singing and removing of clothing.

- The firefighter should speak in short clear phrases: "Get in." "Sit Down." "Wait here."

---

[14] https://www.azcentral.com/story/news/local/...autistic/10601S6001
[15] Cannata, W. (2007). Autism 101 for Fire and Rescue, from SPEAK Website: www.papremisealert.com.

- An individual with autism may take longer to respond to a directive.

- They may not understand what's being demanded of them, or, if scared, may not be able to process the language and understand a directive when fearful.

- When restraint is necessary, be aware that many individuals with autism have a poorly developed upper trunk area. Positional asphyxiation could occur if steps are not taken to prevent it: frequent change of position, not keeping them face down.

- Individuals with autism may continue to resist restraint.

- Children and adults with autism are just as likely to hide in a fire situation. Be sure to check closets, under the bed and behind furniture during a search and rescue.

- These individuals are a bolt risk after rescue.

- It is recommended that firefighters, paramedics or EMTs stay with the individual with autism.[16]

---

[16] *Id.*

Fishers, Indiana (April 2017)

During a recent fire, where it appeared that everyone escaped from the home, rescuers were perplexed why one victim had not escaped like the home's other residents — they could not figure out why the person had not left the building. It was later discovered that the person who was still inside had autism and was more afraid of the lights and sirens than the smoke and flames.

In another fire, a 300-pound man who was brought to safety outside the home, but was so agitated he became violent. The firefighters later found out that he was developmentally disabled and was upset because he left his stuffed bear in the home.

In both of these cases, the firefighters were not informed of crucial information. They only learned that after the fact. Fortunately, both individuals made it to safety. The city of Fishers now has developed a Special Needs Data System. It is a voluntary registry that identifies residents of the community with special needs.

The information — including disability, symptoms, behavior and medication — will appear on a video map during a call, letting first responders know if they need to take extra precautions. The information also could indicate where the victims are most likely to hide, and whether any dangerous items, such as oxygen tanks, are in the home.[17] For this program, people who are bedridden, use a wheelchair and those who are on oxygen are encouraged to register, as well as anyone with a physical or mental disability.[18]

---

[17] John Tuohy, (April 19, 2017) https://www.indystar.com/story/news/2017/04/17/registry-help-fishers-firefighters-rescue-special-needs-victims/100284926/

[18] City of Fishers Special Needs Registry for first responders is designed to help in emergency situations. It can be vitally important for a first responder (a police officer, firefighter, or emergency medical technician) to know that a resident at the address has visual, hearing, mobility, or other special needs; *see* www.fishers.in.us/219/Fishers-Fire-Department. Similarly, Illinois has a state law, since 2009 (the Illinois Premise Alert Program), that requires local governments to start a registry that is kept on a statewide database.

Paramedics and EMTs

Captain Skyler Phillips, EMT-P, of the Chattanooga, Tennessee, Fire Department, has a son with autism. He uses the following *"10 Commandments"* for encountering persons with "special needs" to train other first responders:

(1) Speak directly to the individual (addressing only family or caregivers can be disrespectful).

(2) Shake hands if appropriate.

(3) Identify yourself and your position, which will put them at ease.

(4) Offer assistance and wait for instructions; don't walk up and grab someone's wheelchair.

(5) Treat adults as adults.

(6) Respect wheelchairs and guide dogs.

(7) Listen attentively and ask them to repeat if you don't understand.

(8) Place yourself at eye level; standing over someone is a sign of dominance; face a person who has a hearing impairment.

(9) Relax. Don't be embarrassed to use normal language and phrases.

(10) Assume competence until you know the person's abilities.[19]

Phillips also suggests having available a de-escalation kit for children—such as stickers, coloring books and small toys, snacks, if appropriate, as well as a blanket.

---

[19] https://www.emsworld.com/article/219902/educating-responders-populations-special-needs, also, see Bruce Garner (November 17, 2017) Training First Responders to Respond Better, www.eparent.com/features–3/training-first-responders.

Chapter Five

The Handcuff Dilemma

In recent years, we have witnessed reports of either school resource officers or of other law enforcement officials being called to a school building for an incident involving a young student acting out. In short, the officers decided to handcuff and forcibly restrain the youngsters. The officers have come under tremendous scrutiny for such actions.

> **Kenton County, Kentucky**
>
> In a case in Kenton County, Kentucky, a sheriff's deputy faced a federal lawsuit for handcuffing two elementary school students, ages 8 and 9. A lawsuit was brought by the ACLU, which alleged: there was a unreasonable seizure and excessive force used. The children were handcuffed behind their backs, and the cuffs were place above their elbows because the cuffs would have slipped off of the children's wrists. The video went viral and was made public by the American Civil Liberties Union in 2015.
>
> U.S. District Judge William Bertelsman of the Eastern District of Kentucky ruled that the method the officer used to handcuff the children was "unreasonable and constituted excessive force as a matter of law." During the hearing, the judge noted that the "the video belies" the officer's claim that the cuffs' chain was as wide as the young boy's torso. The judge determined that he would adopt the video as fact over the word of the officer. When the 8-year-old cried out, Bertelsman wrote, it should have been "immediately apparent that this method ... was causing pain." But the boy was left in that position, crying and squirming, for 15 minutes.[20]
>
> The judge noted that a handcuffing expert had testified that he did not know of any police instructor in the United States who would allow the elbow cuffing of children, and that the defense's own handcuffing expert conceded he had

---

[20] https://www.huffingtonpost.com/entry/handcuffs-little-kids-unconstitutional_us_59e127fce4b0a52aca1809ad.

> never trained law enforcement to use handcuffs above the elbow.
>
> "While [the boy] kicked a teacher and [the girl] tried to and/or did hit a teacher, these are very young children, and their conduct does not call to mind the type of 'assault' which would warrant criminal prosecution," Bertelsman wrote. "While Sumner testified that [the boy] swung his elbow towards Sumner, such can hardly be considered a serious physical threat from an unarmed, 54-pound eight-year-old child." [21]
>
> The judge also found that Kenton County was liable for the officer's actions because officials had testified that the handcuffing method was consistent with the policies of the sheriff's office. Sumner had been assigned as a school resource officer by the sheriff's office. [22]
>
> The Civil Rights Division of the U.S. Department of Justice, under then-President Barack Obama, had gotten involved in the lawsuit, arguing that it might not be "objectively reasonable" for a "fully grown man" to handcuff a third-grade boy. DOJ had suggested that the court consider whether the handcuffing was "punitive, rather than necessary to ensure safety," pointing out that the officer had told the child "to behave the way you're supposed to or you suffer the consequences." [23]

When police in St. Petersburg, Florida, handcuffed an unruly 5-year-old kindergartner at Fairmount Park Elementary School, officials had been trying to calm the girl down for more than an hour. The incident was recorded on videotape and aired on television news nationwide.

In the article, "Handcuffing of Children Raises Questions," in *Education Week*, a question was asked, "Is it ever appropriate to handcuff an elementary school pupil?"

---

[21] *Id.*
[22] https://www.huffingtonpost.com/entry/handcuffs-little-kids-unconstitutional_us_59e127fce4b0a52aca1809ad
[23] *Id.*

Randall Marshall, the legal director of the Miami-based Florida chapter of the American Civil Liberties Union, pointed out that the legal system still allows educators to take steps to prevent children from behaving inappropriately. Schools that have ongoing disciplinary problems, he said, need to devote resources to help train staff members and work on disciplinary solutions, rather than rely on police help.[24]

The takeaway: Think twice before restraining a young child with handcuffs. Most law enforcement officials did not receive academy training on how to interact with a child who is acting out. If you are placed in this difficult position, remember that someone will video your encounter and most likely will share it on various social media cites as well as with the news media. *Avoid the use of handcuffs, whenever appropriate.*

The best approach:

- Clear the room of other children who can be hurt, ask the teacher to move the other children out of the room to a safe place.

- Ensure that another adult stays in the room with you (this person could be another teacher or a teacher's assistant). Do not be alone with the child.

- Ask that any and all dangerous objects (scissors, a stapler, long sharp items, rulers, etc.) be removed from the immediate area.

- Sit down, turn the lights off, keep quiet and still (even if the child is yelling and throwing a temper tantrum, let him. As long as the child is safe, yelling and lying on the floor will not hurt them).

- Give the child the time and space to calm down. This is a supervised time out; it may take ten, fifteen or twenty minutes for the child to eventually quiet down. This maneuver is an unexpected one. You are not feeding into the frenzy.

---

[24] https://www.edweek.org/ew/articles/2005/05/18/37handcuffs.h24.html

These are better options than choosing to be the star of an unfortunate handcuffing video.

§5.5. Alzheimer's and Dementia

The *"Silver Tsunami"* is the new metaphor being used to describe the significantly increasing elderly population.

The increasing elderly population will affect health care resources, the economy and the workforce. According to a report published by the government census bureau in March 2018, the nation's Baby Boomer population is largely responsible for this growth.

"The aging of baby boomers means that within just a couple decades, older people are projected to outnumber children for the first time in U.S. history," said Jonathan Vespa, a demographer with the U.S. Census Bureau. "By 2035, there will be 78.0 million people 65 years and older compared to 76.4 million under the age of 18." [25]

As the population ages, the risk factors for Alzheimer's disease, dementia and other age-related diseases increase. According to the research, "[t]he greatest known risk factor for Alzheimer's is increasing age. Most individuals with the disease are 65 and older. After age 65, the risk of Alzheimer's doubles every five years. After age 85, the risk reaches nearly one-third." [26]

Today, there is an estimated 5.7 million Americans of all ages living with Alzheimer's. "This number includes an estimated 5.5 million people age 65 and older and approximately 200,000 individuals under age 65 who have younger-onset Alzheimer's." Moreover, almost "two-thirds of Americans with Alzheimer's are women." [27]

Simply because aging is a risk factor for Alzheimer's disease and dementia does not mean that it is a normal part of aging. It has been determined that a healthy brain may reduce the risk of developing the disease. Simple habits can help keep the brain and body healthy:

---

[25] https://www.census.gov/newsroom/press.../cb18-41-population-projections.html.
[26] https://www.alz.org/alzheimers_disease_causes_risk_factors.asp.
[27] Alzheimer's Facts and Figures Report | Alzheimer's Association https://www.alz.org/facts.

don't smoke, avoid excess alcohol, stay active, eat a healthy diet, and keep the mind and body active.

As the population in the United States ages, law enforcement, firefighters, EMTs, paramedics, and other first responders are increasingly responding to incidents involving older adults. The traditional methods used to control subjects at a scene are often ineffective with these individuals. It is of the utmost importance to find a person with Alzheimer's or dementia within the first 24 hours to ensure their safety and survival. Statistics indicate that after that period of time, the likelihood of finding the person alive is greatly diminished. If a person with Alzheimer's or dementia is reported missing, the "missing persons" protocol should be immediately activated. Here, time is of the essence and an immediate search must be undertaken.

Alzheimer's and dementia are not always apparent, a person may appear physically well, which may be deceiving. There are no obvious physical characteristics. People with the Alzheimer's and related dementia do share many common behaviors and symptoms. Consider the following when searching for a person with the disease.

- They may have an intended destination. They may believe they are going to work, to a store, or to visit someone. Check with their family or a caregiver to determine familiar places for the individual.
- They do not know they are lost or missing.
- They may not answer to hearing their name called. They may not respond to shouts.
- They may not cry out for help.
- They may be near railroad tracks, wooded areas, familiar places and roads, or close to home or bodies of water.
- They may only have traveled less than a few miles from their last location.
- They may be suffering from exposure, disorientation, be dehydrated or dazed and confused.

Response & Assessment - Part I

- They may be fearful of apprehension.
- They may have fallen and unable to stand.

The most common interactions law enforcement officials, firefighters and other first responders may have with older adults with Alzheimer's disease or dementia may be:

- A 911 call that reports wandering by foot or car (most common)
- An auto accident
- False reports to 911
- Shoplifting
- Indecent Exposure
- Getting lost
- Calls for an ambulance
- Victimization
- Suicide
- Criminal complaints
- Elder abuse or neglect
- Request for a welfare check for an older adult
- Home safety
- Taking a car out for a drive without a license
- Gun safety
- Inappropriate behavior in a store or community
- Smell of gas (person forgot to turn off stove)
- Request for fire department

People with Alzheimer's disease or dementia may demonstrate the following behaviors:

- Problems with memory
- Confusion, disorientation
- Hostility and paranoia

- Exhaustion from lack of sleep
- Confusing day and night, or time and place
- Swearing, combative
- Making up stories
- Delusions, irrational
- Inability to answer questions
- May not know how they got somewhere
- May not be able to judge distance
- May accuse others of stealing
- Depression
- Repeating the same thing over and over
- Physical problems, coordination issues, health concerns
- Poor impulse control
- Fearful, anxious
- May not be able to tell you their name or where they live.
- Difficulty completing tasks
- Sundowning—a term used to describe behaviors that intensify in the late afternoon or evening.
- May be unaware of an injury
- No longer understands social conventions or knows appropriate responses
- Wearing inappropriate clothing for the weather

How to interact with a person you suspect or is reported to have Alzheimer's disease or dementia:

Recognize that there may be barriers to communication, such as hearing loss, disorientation, vision impairment, speech difficulty, aphasia (trouble finding the right words to use), and/or cognitive disorders. It is important to distinguish between age-related behaviors associated with dementia and true criminal activity. Always treat the person with dignity; disorientation and memory loss does not mean that they do not perceive disrespect.

Response & Assessment - Part I

    One of the most important things to remember is not to turn your back on the individual or leave them alone, for they could wander away again.

1. First, introduce yourself and verbally state your position.
   Hello, My name is _____.
   I am a _____ (position)
   I am here to help you.
       (Do not assume that they recognize your uniform.)

2. Speak slowly, in a calm reassuring voice.

3. Use specific concrete words.

4. Keep it simple; yes or no questions are best. Ask one thing at a time. Avoid multiple, complex, or wordy instructions.

5. Try to elicit a response that indicates that the person understands. The person may not be able to speak, tell them they can indicate their understanding by nodding their head, moving their hand, etc. Recognize that you may not be able to get a response. The person may have lost the ability to verbally communicate. However, continue to speak to them in a calm, assuring voice. Even if they cannot understand you, your calm tone of voice still serves as a soothing mechanism.

6. You may have to repeat yourself because of the person's short-term memory loss. Be patient.

7. Reassure them that you are there to help.

8. Take your time; you do not want to agitate the individual, which could lead to aggression.

9. Try and keep things calm, if possible reduce loud noises and flashing lights. This will reduce agitation.

10. Do not invade the person's personal space. Getting too close may be perceived as a threat.

11. Explain your actions before proceeding. Avoid physical contact it may appear restraining. If you need to touch them, tell them you will reach for their hand to help them.

12. Recognize that the individual may be uncooperative and combative.

13. The person may not have any memory of what happened.

14. Look for a Medic Alert and/or Safe Return ID jewelry, this could be a bracelet or a necklace. Look for Safe Return Identification.

    The Alzheimer's Association Safe Return® program is a 24-hour nationwide identification, support and enrollment program. They work with law enforcement to quickly identify and return to safety a person with Alzheimer's or a related dementia who has wandered, locally or far from home.

    Also, the Alzheimer's Association and Medic Alert has a nationwide Safe Return Program for people with Alzheimer's and dementia, who wander and become lost. It is a 24-hour emergency response, toll-free hot line (800.625.3780). Located on the person's identification is essential information that identifies the person and will help to reunite the person with their family or caregiver. The service also provides critical medical information to law enforcement and emergency responders. This program may also be used by law enforcement to send an alert to area agencies that a person with Alzheimer's is missing.

15. Provide comfort, a blanket, water, a place to sit (if possible).

16. Observe their physical appearance. Do they have any obvious injuries? Do they wear strong glasses, do they have hearing aids, are they responsive?

17. Depending on the circumstances you may have to listen to their account of the incident or question the individual. In either case, listen and don't interrupt. They may only be able to give you the information one time, they may forget if you interrupt and essential details may be lost.

Response & Assessment - Part I

18. Do not correct them, they believe what they are saying is true. They may perceive situations incorrectly.

19. Do not argue with the person.

20. Do not keep asking the same question if they do not respond, they may not know or be capable of remembering.

21. If appropriate to the situation, ask some or all of the following simple questions to determine their memory and orientation to time and place:

    (A) What is your name?
    (B) Where do you live?
    (C) How old are you?
    (D) When is your birthday?
    (E) What day is it?
    (F) What year is it?
    (G) What month is it?
    (H) Can you count backwards from 10 to 1 for me?
    (I) Who is the President of the United States?

    If they become agitated or upset and cannot answer, back off and stop questioning them. Their actions demonstrate their mental status, and you have your answer. They have some memory impairment.

22. If at all possible, do not use restraints. This may be perceived by the individual as you trying to hurt them, which could escalate into a violent reaction.

23. Find an emergency shelter or help from a social services agency if a family member or caretaker cannot be found.

24. Due to the undetermined nature of the person's condition, many times a first responder or officer will call for an ambulance, especially if the person has no ID and has not been reported as missing. This may be a useful practice, since the person may need medication and evaluation. You may not know how long the individual has been out in the elements and without food or water or their medication. Hospitals have social workers who are equipped with information about resources and support for the

patient and can assist in finding family members and facilities that can assist the individual.

If you are responding to a call where a person with dementia has been accused of shoplifting, a law enforcement presence will make the situation more intense. The person with dementia may become agitated and disoriented. Your first priority should be to calm the situation down. Tell the clerk, store owner or manager that you will deal with the elderly person first, because that is the individual who may be the most volatile. You don't want the person running out of the store and into the street. The situation in the store can wait, that is a stable situation, arrangements for payment or return of the merchandise can be worked out later.

If the person with dementia is agitated, use a calm voice and reassure them. It doesn't matter what the facts are at this point. Your responsibility is to maintain the welfare of the person with Alzheimer's and get them home to a family member or caregiver. You may choose to walk them out of the store and away from the tense scene. Never leave them alone, you don't want them to wander. If you are alone, call for backup.

Listen to the person, no matter what they may be saying. Use phrases such as: "I understand." "I see." "Okay, tell me more." The person believes what they are saying; to them it is the truth, regardless of the true facts. Don't argue, just listen. By allowing them to talk you are defusing the situation and giving them the opportunity to vent. This is very important. If you don't allow them to talk about the incident it may upset and anger them, leading to agitation. At this point you are the person's caretaker until the situation is sorted out. This may take some time, so you will need to be patient. You want a successful outcome, without drama and video recordings. Recognize that once the person is calm and under your supervision, the danger is gone and a successful conclusion may be reached.

San Francisco, July 2017

At an assisted living residence in San Francisco for older adults, Ms. King, an elderly woman with Alzheimer's, grabbed another woman's wrist when she took her seat. No one was injured, and the staff members handled the episode quickly. The woman who had her wrist grabbed also had dementia. She called 911 and said she was attacked. Four officers responded to the call. They decided that Ms. King was unable to care for herself and posed a danger to herself and others. The officers placed the woman under arrest and put her on an involuntary 72-hour psychiatric detention. The officers did not listen to her son and ignored the staff's input about the incident. The woman with Alzheimer's was searched, handcuffed and placed in a patrol car while she was crying.

She was taken to the Psychiatric Emergency Services department at San Francisco General Hospital. At the hospital, the psychiatrist who evaluated Ms. King found her "calm and cooperative" showing no evidence of psychiatric illness, and released her seven hours later.[28] Ms. King's son, Geoffrey, filed a complaint accusing officers of excessive force, unlawful detention and violations of the ADA. "This was such a profound breakdown of procedure and good sense," Geoffrey King said.[29]

In other recent high-profile cases:

- A county sheriff's deputy in Minneapolis, Kansas, used a Taser on a 91-year-old nursing home resident with Alzheimer's who refused to get into a car for a doctor's visit.[30]
- After a 65-year-old in San Jose, California, was arrested and charged with trespassing, a judge — informed that the man had Alzheimer's — dismissed the charge. But deputies at the jail released him before a friend arrived to pick him up, and he wandered onto a highway, and was hit by a car and killed.[31]
- In Bakersfield, California, a 73-year-old man with dementia was walking in his neighborhood late at night

---

[28] https://www.miamiherald.com/news/nation-world/national/article163372383.html.
[29] *Id.*
[30] *Id.*
[31] *Id.*

> when a woman he approached noticed something in his pocket that she thought might have been a gun. When the police arrived and told him to raise his hands, he ignored their shouts, walked toward them, and was shot and killed. The object in his pocket proved to be a crucifix.[32]

Cases such as these demonstrate the critical need for training for law enforcement officials on how to deal with the elderly and people with Alzheimer's and dementia. The elderly may not respond to an officer's command to stop or raise their hands for a variety of reasons. They may not see the person making the request because of poor vision, they may not hear the request, or they may not understand the request due to dementia or another cognitive impairment. If they are told to get down on the ground they may not be able to physically do so.

> **Little Rock, Arkansas, May 2014**
>
> *The headline read:*
>
> > *Man with Alzheimer's Proves That Even If the Mind Forgets, the Heart Remembers*
>
> One day before Mother's Day, police were called when a man with Alzheimer's disease, who had difficulty walking, went missing. His wife, Doris, was frantic. Melvyn Amrine was found wandering two miles from his home. When the police found him, Melyvn had a moment of clarity. He told police that he was looking for a store so he could buy flowers for his wife. Melvyn had been buying his wife flowers for Mother's Day every year since they had their first child. He said he could not go home without flowers.
>
> The two officers were so touched that they stopped at a supermarket and helped Melyvn choose a beautiful bouquet of roses. When Melyvn reached in his pocket he did not have enough money to pay for the flowers. The kind officers gave the cashier the extra cash so Melyvn could buy the flowers.

---

[32] *Id.*

> The officers were quoted as saying that, *"We had to get those flowers, we didn't have a choice."* Doris stood in the doorway when the officers brought her husband of 60 years home. When she saw the flowers she profusely thanked the officers and said, *"It's special, because even though the mind doesn't remember everything, the heart remembers."*[33]

§5.6. Blind and Visually Impaired

According to an October 2017 report from the World Health Organization, the following statistics indicate the number of people worldwide that have some type of vision impairment.

- An estimated 253 million people live with vision impairment: 36 million are blind and 217 million have moderate to severe vision impairment.[34]

- 81% of people who are blind or have moderate or severe vision impairment are aged 50 years and above.[35]

- An estimated 19 million children are vision impaired. Of these, 12 million children have a vision impairment due to refractive error. Around 1.4 million have irreversible blindness, requiring access to vision rehabilitation services to optimize functioning and reduce disability.[36]

> **The Eyes Have It ... Do You See It Now?**
>
> Timmy, a teenage boy who was blind, and intellectually impaired, lost both his eyes at birth. He had glass prosthetic implants that were removable. Timmy enjoyed playing tricks

---

[33] https://www.cbsnews.com/news/as-mans-mind-fades-heart-comes-to-the-rescue/
[34] Bourne RRA, Flaxman SR, Braithwaite T, Cicinelli MV, Das A, Jonas JB, et al.; Vision Loss Expert Group. Magnitude, temporal trends, and projections of the global prevalence of blindness and distance and near vision impairment: a systematic review and meta-analysis. Lancet Glob Health. 2017 Sep;5(9):e888-97
[35] *Id.*
[36] *Id.*

on his teacher. One day, he called out in class, "I'm going to swallow my eye, I'm really gonna do it!" Timmy quickly popped one of his prosthetic eyes out of the socket and put it in his mouth!

As much as his teacher tried to get him to take the glass eye out of his mouth, Timmy wouldn't do it. The teacher watched in horror as Timmy rolled the eyeball around in his mouth. The ball could be seen in his cheek; it looked like a big jawbreaker. Timmy moved the eyeball around and around. He hummed as he moved it from side to side, and up and down. Suddenly, it was gone! The teacher was frantic, 911 was called. When the ambulance arrived, Timmy was placed on the stretcher. The paramedics spoke calmly to Timmy. They looked down his throat, no eye! The teacher kept asking, do you see it now? Timmy then reached in his pants pocket and pulled out his eye and asked, "Do you see it now?"

This is a true story; the author was the boy's teacher. The boy's name was changed. It was a good thing that the paramedics were calm and comforting to the boy, who ultimately cooperated.

When interacting with a person who is blind or visually impaired:

- Always verbally identify yourself when approaching a blind or visually impaired person.

- Since the person doesn't see you, it is necessary for you to provide information to the individual; such as your name, your badge number or other identifying information.

- Recognize that many times, persons who are blind have been victims of people impersonating public officials, therefore, a request to feel your badge will provide a level of assurance to the person that you are indeed an officer. If you have a radio you may need to contact someone at headquarters or dispatch to verify your identity. Again, this a reasonable

Response & Assessment - Part I

accommodation that can be met to assure the individual of your identity.

- Keep in mind that nothing that is visual and obvious to you is seen by the person who is blind.

- Inform the person of anything in the environment that may be an obstacle. Remember, they may be upset, frightened and disoriented at this point.

- Ask the person if they need assistance before touching or physically guiding them. You don't want to startle them. If they do ask you for assistance, ask them how they want to be helped.

- If you are guiding the individual verbally, use specific terms and directions, such as: straight in front of you, to your right there is a handrail, we will take three steps down.

- Depending on the circumstances, you may have to listen to their account of the incident or question the individual. In either case, listen and don't interrupt.

- Do not discount what they have to say because they are blind or visually impaired. They may have pertinent information to offer.

- Tell them what will happen before you do it. This is very important. Since they can't see you, telling the person what you will do before you do it will provide assurance.

- Monitor *how* you speak to the individual, *don't talk down* to the person.

- Speak directly to the individual, *don't talk about them* to others in front of them. This could be perceived as condescending and rude.

- Don't shout, you may ask them if they can hear you, that's acceptable.

- Let the person know if you have a partner with you. If someone else arrives at or leaves the scene inform them.

- Provide comfort, a blanket, water, a place to sit if possible.

- If this is a domestic violence call, the person with the disability may be the one who is hurt, you may have to separate the individuals to determine the facts. Recognize that the caregiver or family member may be the perpetrator. And, as in other domestic violence situations, the individual may be fearful of talking in front of the caregiver or other family member.

If the person who is blind has a specialized cane, do not take it away. The cane is protected and recognized as an assistive device by the Americans with Disabilities Act, as well as Section 504 of the Rehabilitation Act.

Service Animals

If the person has a service animal, it also is a protected class under the Americans with Disabilities Act and Section 504 of the Rehabilitation Act. You must respond appropriately to someone using a service animal. Do not take the dog away. It is not considered a "pet." Do not touch the service animal when they are working.

The ADA defines a service dog as one that is trained to perform "work or tasks" in the aid of a disabled person. A true service dog maintains the health and welfare of its human partner. A true service dog is a specially trained large breed dog, usually a German Shepard, a Labrador Retriever, or a Golden Retriever. There are also seizure alert dogs that have been trained to respond and assist people with epilepsy. Service animals may also be used for people with disabilities, such as hearing loss, and diabetic individuals; they are intended for people with a disability.

Service dogs are now being trained to work with veterans who have post-traumatic stress and other severe disabilities. The task(s) performed by the dog must directly relate to the person's disability.

Response & Assessment - Part I

According to ada.gov, there are only two questions that can be asked to determine if a dog is a service animal, they are:

> In situations where it is not obvious that the dog is a service animal, staff may ask only two specific questions: (1) is the dog a service animal required because of a disability? and (2) what work or task has the dog been trained to perform? Staff are not allowed to request any documentation for the dog, require that the dog demonstrate its task, or inquire about the nature of the person's disability.[37]

Terminology

The language and terms that describe various types of working animals or animals that help people with disabilities are not consistently used or understood. When different people say "service animal," "assistance animal," "comfort animal," "emotional support animal," or "therapy animal," they are not necessarily talking about the same thing.[38]

The topic of service animals and other types of animals that help people with disabilities has become nearly too hot to handle in recent years. This is an area where multiple laws, which sometimes overlap, apply in various settings.[39]

Emotional Support and Comfort Animals

There is a great deal of confusion with the "in vogue" use of "emotional support" or "comfort" animals. These animals are not trained to perform specific disability-related tasks. They provide passive benefit; their presence is comforting to their owner. They are everywhere, and there is now a sense of entitlement owners have for taking their cute pets into eating establishments, markets and stores. These pets are not service animals. Only true service animals are permitted in all establishments. Individual states can determine the guidelines for emotional support pets in their communities. For

---

[37] https://www.ada.gov/regs2010/service_animal_qa.html.
[38] http://www.adainfo.org/content/service-animals, Fall 2015.
[39] *Id.*

example, in Florida, the person may be required to provide a letter from his or her medical provider that (1) indicates that the patient is currently under the medical provider's care; (2) references the mental impairment that substantially affects one or more enumerated life activities; and (3) provides a medical opinion that the animal provides emotional support that alleviates one or more identified symptoms or effects of the patient's existing disability.

Therapy Animals

Therapy animals are trained by handlers and taken to various places such as hospitals, nursing homes, schools, and other places to provide therapeutic benefits for many people. We have seen them taken to places after a terrible tragedy to provide comfort to traumatized people. These animals are working animals but do not meet the ADA definition of a service animal because they do not serve one person with a disability.

Assistance Animals

The United States Department of Housing and Urban Development uses the term Assistance Animals in relation to the Fair Housing Act (FHA) as well as Section 504 of the Rehabilitation Act. It can include animals of various types that perform tasks or provide emotional support for individuals with disabilities.

Under Title II and Title III, only dogs can be considered a service animal. In 2010, the Department of Justice revised their definition and eliminated the "other animal" part of the law. A service animal can be any type, size, or breed of dog.

> *Cats, monkeys, goats, rats, snakes, rabbits, pigs, or other types of animals, regardless of whether they have been trained to perform tasks for people with disabilities or how well-behaved they might be, are not considered service animals under DOJ's rules.*[40]

NOTE: If you have concerns or questions about the use of a cane for the blind or the use of a service animal at a scene, before taking any action, it would be advisable to contact your agency's legal

---

[40] http://www.adainfo.org/content/service-animals.

Response & Assessment - Part I

advisor, prosecutor, district attorney, or your agency's special needs liaison. Most important, your agency should have specific policies in place to determine beforehand what actions should be taken in these circumstances.

In such cases, it would be best to ask yourself the following:

- Is a full custodial arrest really necessary?

- Can the situation best be served by issuing a summons instead of handcuffing the person and transporting them to headquarters?

- Is this situation so critical or urgent that there is eminent harm?

- Will this incident garner unfavorable media attention, harming the reputation of the officer and his or her agency?

§5.7. Deafness and Hearing Impairment

According to a March 2018 report from the World Health Organization the following statistics indicate the number of people worldwide that have some type of disabling hearing loss.

- Around 466 million people worldwide have disabling hearing loss, 34 million of these are children.

- It is estimated that by 2050, over 900 million people will have disabling hearing loss.

- Hearing loss may result from genetic causes, complications at birth, certain infectious diseases, chronic ear infections, the use of particular drugs, exposure to excessive noise, and aging.

- 60% of childhood hearing loss is due to preventable causes.

- 1.1 billion young people (aged between 12–35 years) are at risk of hearing loss due to exposure to noise in recreational settings.

- Unaddressed hearing loss poses an annual global cost of $750 billion. Interventions to prevent, identify and address hearing loss are cost-effective and can bring great benefit to individuals.

- People with hearing loss benefit from early identification; use of hearing aids, cochlear implants and other assistive devices; captioning and sign language; and other forms of educational and social support.[41]

The functional impact of hearing loss is the person's ability to communicate. The causes of hearing loss and deafness may be either congenital or acquired at a later age. The loss may be mild, moderate or severe, as well as total deafness.

Under the Americans with Disabilities Act people who are deaf or hard of hearing are entitled to the same services as anyone else. "Law enforcement agencies must make efforts to ensure that their personnel communicate effectively with people whose disability affects hearing. This applies to both sworn and civilian personnel."[42]

When an agency needs an interpreter for the person who is deaf the agency cannot charge for this service. If an interpreter is needed for official communication, such as a statement, it should be an impartial, qualified or licensed interpreter (not a family member). In these situations, a relative or caregiver would be inappropriate because they have emotional ties and may not be impartial. Nonetheless, a family member could be used when it is an urgent need, such as an accident or medical emergency.

---

[41] https://www.who.int/news-room/fact-sheets/detail/deafness-and-hearing-loss.
[42] https://www.ada.gov/lawenfcomm.htm.,January 2006.

Response & Assessment - Part I

It is not appropriate to ask a person who is deaf to pay for or provide an interpreter, which is the agencies responsibility. An interpreter may be needed when interviewing a witness, a suspect or an arrestee.

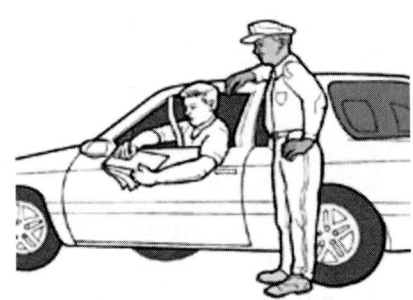

A driver who is deaf writes on a pad of paper to communicate with an officer.*
*www.ada.gov/lawenfcomm.htm.January2006.

Example: An officer clocks a car on the highway going 15 miles per hour above the speed limit. The driver, who is deaf, is pulled over and is issued a noncriminal citation. The individual is able to understand the reason for the citation because the officer points out relevant information printed on the citation or written by the officer.[43]

The most critical moments people who are deaf have with law enforcement officers are in the first moments before the official realizes that the person is deaf. First contact is the most important stage of the interaction. This is the moment when the person who is deaf may reach in a pocket for deaf ID or a pad and pencil, but the officer believes the person is reaching for a weapon; or the deaf person does not respond to verbal directions and the officer may believe the person is noncompliant.

It would be best during a traffic stop if the individual who is deaf had a deaf ID on the driver's side window. Until this happens, officers will have to be very careful when interacting with drivers who are deaf.

When interacting with a person who is deaf or hearing impaired:

- Do not touch their head or their ears. The person may have hearing aids that could be dislodged. They could also have a cochlear implant.

---

[43] *Id.*

- Do not restrict their hands, this is their method of communicating.

- Have a paper and a pen available to communicate by writing.

- If they are wearing hearing aids, do not assume that they will hear everything you say. Hearing aids amplify sounds, but can also amplify noise, if there is ambient noise in the area, the individual may not be able to hear your words and what you are saving. Have a pen and paper as backup for written communication.

- Don't raise your voice or shout, speaking louder will not help.

- If the person reads lips, speak normally. Make sure you are in a well-lighted area.

- Don't chew gum or have anything in your mouth. This distorts your lip movements, thereby hampering the person's ability to read your lips.

- Face the person so they can see your face and lips.

- Minimize background noise and other distractions.

- Before speaking make sure you have the person's attention.

- Use visual aids if possible, point to written information.

- A person who has ear buds in their ears and listening to an electronic device may not be hearing impaired but may not hear you.

- If the person asks for an interpreter you must comply, which is a reasonable accommodation and required as part of the Americans with Disabilities Act (ADA) and Section 504 of the Rehabilitation Act. Make sure you ask which language the person uses, the most common are American Sign Language (ASL) or Signed English.

- Serious consideration should be given before handcuffs are used. If absolutely necessary, handcuff the person from the front, not from behind. Since their hands are their communication tool, this accommodation is essential.

> **Aurora, Colorado, August 2, 2018**
>
> Gary Black, a 73-year-old veteran who was the recipient of a Bronze Star and the Purple Heart, was fatally shot by police after killing a violent intruder in his home. The man had "significant" hearing loss sustained during his time in the military and may not have heard the officer's commands to drop his gun. The family was asleep in their home, when a naked intruder (who had been at a party across the street) kicked in the door, ripping it off the hinges. The intruder dragged the vet's 11-year-old grandson into the bathroom where he violently attacked the boy and tried to drown him. Black and his stepson tried to stop the attacker. Black then reportedly got his gun and shot the intruder in the chest, killing him. At some point, Black's wife called 911. The officers who responded saw Black with a gun inside and opened fire, killing him.[44]
>
> It was reported that officers heard Black's wife say, "He has a gun" before encountering the Vietnam veteran holding a firearm and a flashlight. The officers ordered Black to drop the gun and show his hands, but he didn't comply. Black was walking toward the officers and raising the flashlight, still holding the gun, when one opened fire, fatally wounding him. The officers later found the intruder, dead in the bathroom. The intruder had violently assaulted Black's grandson before being killed. Police said the intruder didn't know the family and it appears to have been a random assault. The grandson was taken to the hospital for serious, non–life-threatening issues.[45]
>
> The officer who fired the shot has been placed on administrative reassignment with pay, according to the Denver

---

[44] https://www.nbcnews.com/.../police-describe-chaotic-scene-veteran-killed-after-self-de...
[45] https://taskandpurpose.com/army-veteran-police-naked-intruder/

Post, and the 17th Judicial District Attorney's Office and *Denver Police* are investigating.

Oklahoma City, September 2017

A man who was deaf and developmentally disabled was fatally shot in front of his own home when he did not respond to the commands to stop and drop. The police had been called because of a "hit and run" accident in the street in front of the man's home. Upon arrival at around 8:15 p.m., an officer saw Magdiel Sanchez, 35, holding a 2-foot-long metal pipe "wrapped in some type of material" with a small leather loop on the end of it. A neighbor had later stated that Sanchez often carried the pipe to fend off stray dogs when he went for walks at night. When the officer saw the pipe, he called for backup since he perceived it as a weapon.

Sanchez, who was deaf, was not involved in the hit and run but was on his porch. When another police unit arrived, verbal commands were being given to Sanchez to "drop the weapon and get on the ground." According to the report, just before the shooting, witnesses yelled, "he can't hear you, he's deaf." When Sanchez allegedly advanced toward the officers, they Tasered and shot him. According to the autopsy report, Sanchez was killed when he was shot five times in front of his home—he could not hear the command to stop.[46]

The officers who shot and tasered Sanchez did not have body cameras. The department is in the process of getting them. The police spokesperson stated that he did not know why officers didn't respond to neighbors' warnings that Sanchez was deaf.

---

[46] https://www.nbcnews.com/.../deaf-man-shot-dead-oklahoma-city-police-neighbors-scr...

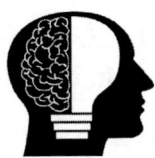

KEY POINTS

- The officer's job is not to diagnosis, but to observe, access and to determine if a person may have special needs and modify your response accordingly.

- Just because a person has a disability does not mean that they are not dangerous. Always guard your weapons and be alert until you determine the threat assessment.

- The rate of violent victimization against persons with disabilities was 2.5 times higher than the rate for persons without disabilities.

- It is more likely that a law enforcement officer, firefighter or other first responder will be called to scene where a person with a disability may be the victim of a crime rather than the perpetrator of the crime.

- The drug epidemic has had a serious impact on the law enforcement officials, firefighters, and other first responders. Not surprisingly, because of this, the number of calls to 911 have significantly increased.

- The drug epidemic has presented new risks to the first responders. Exposure to drug paraphernalia, fentanyl and its derivatives, as well as other drugs poses a threat to anyone responding to the scene.

- Fentanyl can be ingested orally, inhaled through the nose or mouth, or absorbed through the skin or eyes, any substance suspected to contain fentanyl should be treated with extreme caution.

- The CDC reports that 1 out of 59 children (1 in 37 boys and 1 in 151 girls) have been identified as having an Autism Spectrum Disorder. Autism is 4 times more common in boys than girls.

KEY POINTS (Continued)

- A person with autism might demonstrate certain behaviors and characteristics and react in an inappropriate manner. For example, they may:
  - ~ wander; they may be unable to understand danger.
  - ~ be overwhelmed by flashing lights, certain sounds, loud noises, sirens, or fire.
  - ~ be afraid of a person in uniform, or a firefighter in turnout gear.
  - ~ demonstrate curiosity and reach for objects or equipment such as a shiny badge or handcuffs or even your gun.
  - ~ not respond or understand commands such as stop or put your hands up.
  - ~ not speak, may not respond to his or her name.
  - ~ display repetitive behaviors known as stimming by rocking back and forth, hand flapping, hitting himself, head rolling, spinning, or other similar behaviors.
  - ~ not respond to pain in a typical way and may not be able to explain their pain.
- If there are people around who know the autistic person, listen to what they say. They may have important information about this individual.
- When responding to calls involving subjects with autism, the majority of those times, you will be handling a person in crisis, not a criminal.
- Think twice before restraining a young child with handcuffs.
- Today, there is an estimated 5.7 million Americans of all ages living with Alzheimer's dementia.

Response & Assessment - Part I

KEY POINTS (Continued)

- It is of the utmost importance to find a person with Alzheimer's or dementia within the first 24 hours to ensure their safety and survival. Statistics indicate that after that period of time, the likelihood of finding the person alive is greatly diminished.

- The most common interactions law enforcement officials, firefighters and other first responders may have with older adults with Alzheimer's disease or dementia may be a 911 call that reports wandering by foot or car (most common); an auto accident; false reports to 911; shoplifting; or indecent exposure.

- People with Alzheimer's disease or dementia may demonstrate: problems with memory, confusion, disorientation, hostility, paranoia, exhaustion or delusions.

- When interacting with a person who is blind or visually impaired, always verbally identify yourself; since the person doesn't see you, it is necessary for you to provide information to the individual, such as your name, your badge number or other identifying information.

- When interacting with a person who is blind, ask the person if they need assistance before touching or physically guiding them. You don't want to startle them. If they do ask you for assistance, ask them how they want to be helped.

- If the person has a service animal, it also is a protected class under the law; it is not a pet; do not touch the service animal when it is working.

- The functional impact of hearing loss is the person's ability to communicate.

- When interacting with a person who is deaf or hearing impaired:
    - Do not touch the head or ears of a person who is hearing impaired. The person may have hearing aids that could be dislodged. The person could also have a cochlear implant.
    - Do not restrict their hands, this is their method of communicating.

KEY POINTS (Continued)

- Have paper and a pen available to communicate by writing for someone who is hearing impaired.
- Don't raise your voice or shout, speaking louder will not help.
- If the person reads lips, speak normally. Make sure you are in a well-lighted area.
- Minimize background noise and other distractions.
- Use visual aids if possible, point to written information.

Chapter Six
RESPONSE & ASSESSMENT – PART II

§6.1. Mental Illness

As identified in previous chapters, the Centers for Disease Control (CDC) reports that mental illnesses are among the most common health conditions in the United States. Negative attitudes and misconceptions associated with mental health and mental illness still exist. The following facts demonstrate the statistics of mental illness in the United States.

- In 2016, there were 44.7 million adults—about 1 in 5 Americans—with a mental illness.[1]

- In 2016, there were an estimated 10.4 million adults with serious mental illness. This represents 4.2% of all U.S. adults.[2]

- Just over 20%—or 1 in 5—children have had a serious debilitating mental disorder.[3]

- Half of all chronic mental illness begins by age 14 and three-quarters begin by age 24.[4]

- Suicide, which is often associated with symptoms of mental illness, is the tenth leading cause of death in the United States and the second leading cause of death among people aged 19 to 34.[5]

---

[1] https://www.nimh.nih.gov//health/topics/index.shtml. Data presented from 2016 National Survey on Drug Use and Health(NSDUH)by the Substance Abuse and Mental Health Services Administration (SAMHSA).
[2] Id.
[3] Health & Education Statistics (http://www.nimh.nih.gov/health/statistics/prevalence/
[4] Id.
[5] Rui P, Hing E, Okeyode T. National Ambulatory Medical Care Survey: 2014 State and National Summary Tables. Atlanta, GA: National Center for Health Statistics. Centers for Disease Control and Prevention. 2014.

These statistics speak for themselves. Consequently, the likelihood of a law enforcement officer, firefighter, EMT, paramedic, or other first responder encountering someone with a mental illness is high. Recognizing these individuals is important, yet their impairment is very difficult to determine quickly. There is no single cause for mental illness.

Mental illness should not be confused with cognitive impairment. They are two different things. People who have mental illness usually have average or above-average intelligence but have difficulty functioning in their daily lives because of the illness. On the other hand, cognitive impairment can refer to numerous conditions that can impact learning, communication, processing, and remembering. Cognitive impairment may be mild, moderate or severe, and will be addressed later on in this chapter. This section is specific to mental illness.

The study of mental illness has evolved over the years, but no one can exactly predict the behavior of others. Dealing with a person with a mental illness wielding a gun is serious and unpredictable. The media can overly simplify news by sensationalizing events. One of the negative outcomes of this is the belief that many individuals that are mentally ill frequently engage in violent behavior. Yet studies show that the majority of individuals with mental illness are never violent.

Mental illness is strongly associated with increased risk of suicide, which accounts for over half of the firearms-related fatalities in the United States. People who have mental illness may be your neighbor, a coworker, a friend, a family member, or almost anyone you encounter. Many people with a mental illness manage to live their lives and function with the help of medical professionals. They live their lives without harming others and we may not even be aware of their conditions. Those individuals that have serious mental issues cannot function well. Statistics indicate that 10.4 million adults, 4.2% of the United States adult population lives with serious mental health issues.

In Chapter One, an explanation of how the deinstitutionalization policy, which began in the mid 1950s, had a tremendous effect on the mental health crisis in the United States. Many experts have determined that this policy did not work. The direct effect has been experienced on a daily basis by law enforcement officials, firefighters, EMTs, paramedics, and other first responders across the country. These are the individuals that make up part of the homeless population; some may be seriously mentally ill; some may be veterans, indigents, or the hopeless. They are seen on the streets of America every day.

By itself, mental illness does not predict violence, "but having a mental illness and a substance abuse problem [does] increase the risk of violence."[6]

The symptoms that categorize mental illness may be vast, some are easily identifiable and observable, whereas others may be more difficult. You are not expected to be able to diagnose these problems, rather, you may be able to recognize some of the behavioral warning signs. One of the most difficult and pressing issues is how to get help for someone with a mental illness that doesn't accept assistance or refuses the help.[7]

A dangerous situation can occur when individuals with mental illnesses may provoke police into killing them. This is now commonly known as "suicide by cop" (SBC). The term "SBC" was "coined in 1983 by Karl Harris, a Los Angeles County medical examiner."[8] In Arizona, the following is an excerpt from a story in a local newspaper:

> **Suicide-by-Cop**
>
> *A despondent man was fatally shot Saturday by Phoenix police in what authorities said may be a case of suicide by cop .... During nearly 40 minutes of negotiations, [a spokesperson] said, the obviously despondent driver repeatedly aimed the weapon at his head. Eventually, he stepped out of the car and pointed the weapon*

---

[6] https://www.psychologytoday.com/...management/.../communicating-people-mental-il...
[7] *Id.*
[8] https://www.mdedge.com/.../suicide-cop-what-motivates-those-who-choose-method.

> at his head, then took aim at police, she said. Five officers opened fire, mortally wounding the man."[9]

In Nevada, a man called 911 and warned of his plans for suicide by cop:

> *Las Vegas police officers killed a man early Wednesday after he reached for what they believed was a gun .... The victim, whose identity was withheld pending notification of his relatives, called 911 and told a dispatcher he wanted police officers to kill him, police said .... The officers called a crisis intervention officer to talk to the victim without any luck. The officers then got within 20 feet of the man and shot him with a Taser gun in an attempt to subdue him without injury. The Taser temporarily incapacitated him. However, once the electrical charge from the device wore off, the man reached for his waistband and pulled out what police believed was a gun, police said. At that point, three of the four officers present opened fire and shot the man several times. The man was pronounced dead at University Medical Center."*[10]

When a mentally ill person decides to initiate a "suicide by cop" incident, they must have premeditated a well-thought out plan. This event is not an accident, but a plan that has a beginning, a middle and a deadly end:

1. The suicidal person creates an event that would ensure police response.

2. Once the officers arrive at the scene, the person begins aggressive actions forcing a confrontation.

3. The person tells the officers that they have a weapon.

---

[9] https://mentalillnesspolicy.org/crimjust/law-enforcement-mental-illness.html.
[10] https://mentalillnesspolicy.org/crimjust/law-enforcement-mental-illness.html.

4. The person may threaten the officers, may sometimes injure an officer or other citizen to increase the lethality and urgency of the situation.

5. The person refuses to surrender and may express his desire to be killed by officers.

6. The person walks or runs toward the officers and refuses to drop his weapon forcing the officers to engage.[11]

In situations such as this, experts have suggested a Crisis Response Team, who are officers who have training in handling individuals with the psychiatric disorders of mental illness, to be established so that they may be dispatched in these circumstances.

In the article, *Suicide By Cop: What motivates those who choose this method?*, Doctors Similien and Okorafor discuss the issues that may lead a person to choose this method of suicide. They note that the individual may choose this method to avoid the shameful consequences of killing oneself, to avoid the exclusions from life insurance policies so that their families may collect the benefits, and may rationalize that it avoids the religious and spiritual tenets against suicide, thereby saving face.[12] Or the person may use the confrontation with the police to communicate hopelessness, depression, or desperation.

SBC accounts for 10% to 36% of police shootings and can cause serious stress for the officers involved. It certainly can create a strain between the police and the community.[13] Always use extreme care in situations where mental illness is a factor. Things can go from bad to worse in a matter of seconds. It is critical to have backup when dealing with a person with mental illness. Do not assume that a small person can be managed alone. An individual can have tremendous strength once their adrenaline starts to flow, and may be able to inflict significant harm.

---

[11] Lester D. Suicide as a staged performance. Comprehensive Psychology. 2015:4(1):1-6.
[12] https://www.mdedge.com/psychiatry/article/136342/depression/suicide-cop-what-motivates-those-who-choose-method.
[13] *Id.*

Some Characteristics of Mental Illness:

- inappropriate responses
- a lack of response is also notable
- extreme hyperactivity
- laughing at a serious event
- talking but making no sense
- hallucinations, hearing voices, seeing things that are not there
- delusions, paranoia
- serious functional impairment in activities of daily living
- staring into space
- anxiety, panic, fright
- unaware of passing time
- inability to make eye contact
- unresponsive to questions yet the person can hear you
- inability to focus on any task
- depressed
- excessive sleep, tiredness, problems sleeping
- confused thinking
- extreme mood changes, highs and lows
- withdrawal
- excessive emotions, such as anger, hostility or violence
- alcohol or drug abuse
- unable to cope with normal life
- suicidal thoughts

Effective methods for interacting with people who have mental illness is outlined below.

- An officer should not handle a person suspected as having a mental illness alone. If you are sent to a scene and suspect that the person has a mental illness, call and wait for backup.

- Approach the individual in a calm, non-threatening manner.

- Do not get too close, give the person some space, don't touch the individual. You do not want to appear threatening.

- Introduce yourself and be respectful.

Response & Assessment – Part II

- Recognize that the person may be frightened by you, they may be unable to determine if you are there to help or hurt them.

- Recognize that the person may be overwhelmed, scared and having delusions, which makes them even more unstable.

- Keep it simple, use simple sentences and speak slowly.

- Use appropriate language, don't use negative words such as nutcase, crazy, etc.

- Give the person time to process and respond.

- You may have to repeat your statement.

- Don't raise your voice or shout.

- Try to gather some identifying information from the individual.

- If possible, determine if the person has a caregiver or family member, and contact them.

- Do not discount what they have to say because they appear mentally ill. They may have pertinent information to offer.

- Unless the circumstances dictate otherwise, tell them what you plan to do before you do it. This is very important. Since they may be disoriented and or frightened, telling the person what you will do before you do it will provide the individual with some sense of safety.

- Monitor how you speak to the individual, don't talk down to the person.

- Speak directly to the individual, don't talk about them to others in front of them. This could be perceived as condescending and rude.

- Avoid sudden movements.

- Don't joke with the person, they may interpret it incorrectly.

- If the individual is acting out, or uncontrollable, the person may be in crisis and needs immediate intervention. In this situation immediately contact a mental health crisis center or call for an ambulance to take the person to a hospital.

- Determine if the person is injured. If that is the case, call an ambulance immediately. The individual may not be able to explain their injury and may be more seriously injured than what is apparent.

- Don't disagree with the individual, they may be having delusions or hallucinations and believe something to be true. This may be frightening to the person. Just assure the person that you are there to protect them.

- If the person is noncommunicative, don't continue to ask questions. Don't assume that the individual does not hear you, they may hear you and cannot or will not respond. Call mental health services for assistance.

- If the person threatens suicide take it seriously.

- Since a person with a severe mental illness may try to hurt themselves in your presence, be sure to keep your gun secure.

- Be aware that the individual may try to bite, head butt, kick, or spit.

- The person with a mental illness does not have typical responses, they may appear calm and manageable at first and be uncontrollable in the next second.

- Persons with mental illness who have been victimized may have a more extreme response to the event.

- Very serious consideration should be given to any situation that would require an arrest. Due to the volatile situation, you do not have a satisfactory assessment of the person's physical condition. Things can spiral out of control very quickly with this person. Extreme caution is advised.

- Since you are unaware of the extent of the mental illness, the type of prescription drugs the person may be taking, and whether the person is taking any illegal drugs or alcohol, your best option may be to call for an ambulance.

- Recognize that making the decision to use medical transport provides the best chance for the safety of the person with mental illness and the public safety officials on the scene. Transporting the person in a patrol car or police van may be a bad idea.

§6.2. Intellectual Disability

A person with an intellectual disability has sub-average general intellectual functioning, along with deficits in both cognitive capacity and adaptive behavior. An intellectual disability does not have a specific age requirement, but the symptoms begin during the developmental period of childhood. It is characterized by limitations in reasoning, learning, problem solving and adaptive behavior. It is a lifelong disorder that impacts everyday life. It may range from mild to moderate, or in the most serious cases, severe to profound. The test that determines this disability is known as an IQ Test.

An intellectual disability is not the same as a developmental disability. A developmental disability may include an intellectual disability but also includes physical disabilities. A person might have both disabilities or may have either one.

There is a great deal of history and some negativity against the use of IQ Tests to determine intelligence. Society places extreme importance on intellectual abilities. As explained in Chapter One, the eugenics movement began in the United States in the early 1900s. The goal was to improve the physical, mental and emotional genetics of the family, thereby limiting the negative traits through careful selection and breeding. Twenty-nine states enacted sterilization laws, which unfortunately found legal support in the 1927 Supreme Court decision of *Buck v. Bell*.[14]

In that case, speaking for the Supreme Court, Justice Oliver Wendell Holmes opined, "It is better for all the world, if instead of waiting to execute degenerate offspring for crime, or to let them starve for imbecility, society can prevent those who are manifestly unfit from continuing their kind …. Three generations of imbeciles are enough."[15]

This Supreme Court decision legitimized the various sterilization laws in the United States. Over 65,000 people were sterilized. In particular, California's program was so robust that the Nazis turned to California for advice in perfecting their own efforts. Hitler proudly admitted to following the laws of several American states that allowed for the prevention of reproduction of the "unfit."[16] For a more in-depth review of this topic refer to Chapter Four.

Eventually, the use of the offensive words, feebleminded and imbeciles, was replaced with the term "mental retardation." Today, the term "mentally retarded" is no longer used, and has been replaced with the term "intellectual disability." This demonstrates the continued search for a description that is less offensive. An intellectual disability is determined by using approved standardized tests, which generate an IQ score. Medical evaluations may also be useful in this determination.

A person's Intelligence Quotient — one's **IQ** — is a statistical score determined by standardized tests used to measure human intelligence. However, it measures only specific aspects and is not the truest measure of someone's intellectual capacity. There are multiple IQ tests comprised of questions in the areas of verbal and performance that measure general knowledge, language, reasoning,

---

[14] 274 U.S. 200 (1927).
[15] *Buck v. Bell*, 274 U.S. 200, 207 (1927); *see also* Black, Edwin, *"The Horrifying American Roots of Nazi Eugenics."* History News Network. N.p., Sept. 2003. Web. 07 May 2014. <http://hnn.us/article/1796>.
[16] https://www.nature.com/.../america-s-hidden-history-the-eugenics-movement-12391944...

memory skills, conceptual skills, spatial, sequencing and problem-solving skills. These tests produce scores that are considered estimates of intelligence. Such exams do not, however, measure everything. There are two types of intelligence that cannot be measured in the standard IQ test: "Emotional Intelligence" (EQ) and "Social Intelligence" (SQ). Some experts believe that one's EQ is more important than IQ. This has been, and will continue to be, a hot topic.

According to *Psychology Today*, Social Intelligence "develops from experience with people and learning from success and failures in social settings. It is more commonly referred to as 'tact,' 'common sense' or 'street smarts.'" [17]

In contrast, having Emotional Intelligence is having "the ability to identify and manage your own emotions and the emotions of others." [18] The skill requires the person to utilize emotion in problem solving and thinking.

Ludwig Wilhelm Stern, a German psychologist and philosopher, described as a pioneer in personality and intelligence, coined the term, intelligence quotient, in 1912. That term was later used by an American psychologist, who worked for the U.S. Army, by the name of Lewis Madison Terman. He further developed the intelligence quotient in 1916. The first mass IQ tests were given to U.S. soldiers during World War I. [19]

According to Terman's scale, anyone with a score under 70 is classified as "definite feebleminded"; anyone with a score between 70 and 79, would have "borderline deficiency"; anyone with a score between 80-89 would be afflicted with "dullness." Most people have a score between 90 and 109, which means that they are classed as having a normal or average intelligence. Once you get an IQ score of 110 you begin to take note. A score between 110 and 119 would indicate a superior intelligence; a score between 120 and 140 would

---

[17] https://www.ie.edu/.../social-intelligence-vs-emotional-intelligence-making-distinction-...
[18] *Id.*
[19] https://sciencetrends.com/highest-possible-iq-people-hold-world-record/

mean a very superior intelligence; a score over 140 would indicate genius or near genius." [20]

A standard deviation, which has been determined to be 15 points, is possible on any IQ test, this means that a **plus (+) or minus (-) of a 15-point** variation is possible in either direction. When IQ tests were first developed, the mean was established at 100. This means that the average normal IQ is 100. If you're below 100, you're less intelligent than average and above 100 the opposite (note that is just for this test). The IQ score moves 15 points in either direction with each standard deviation. [21]

One must recognize that giftedness and genius may be found in any field, mathematics, music, sports, computer science, physics, art, or medicine, just to name a few. "One of America's greatest inventive geniuses: Thomas Alva Edison, like Einstein, was not a very good student, and quite likely would not have scored very high on an IQ test in childhood. But Edison, like all geniuses of great accomplishment, had boundless drive, and understood perfectly the essence of genius when he wrote, "Genius is one percent inspiration and 99 percent perspiration." [22]

The basic range of Intelligence Quotient (IQ) scores are as follows:

- 69 and below: Intellectual Disability
- 70 to 79:   Borderline Intellectual Disability
- 80 to 89:   Low Average Range
- 90 to 109:   Normal Intelligence Range
- 110 to 119:   High Average Range
- 120 to 129:   Gifted/Superior Range
- 130+:   Very Superior Range
- 140+:   Genius IQ Range

---

[20] *Id.*
[21] https://sciencetrends.com/highest-possible-iq-people-hold-world-record/
[22] https://www.Genuis: An Overview, William, E. Benet, Ph.D., Psy.D., January, 2005. assessmentpsychology.com.

There is even a society dedicated to people with superior intelligence. Mensa International is the oldest high IQ society in the world. To qualify for membership, you must score at the 98th percentile on a supervised, and standardized, approved IQ test. The minimum score that is accepted by Mensa is 131.

What are some of the highest IQ scores ever recorded?[23]

- Stephen Hawking (IQ score – 160)
    (theoretical physicist)

- Albert Einstein (IQ score – 160 – 190)
    (Nobel Prize winning scientist)

- Judit Polgar (IQ score – 170)
    (youngest chess grandmaster at 15 years old)

- Philip Emeagwali (IQ score – 190)
    (mathematician, computer scientist, engineer)

- Garry Kasparov (IQ score – 194)
    (chess master, ranked No. One 225 times)

- Christopher Langan (IQ score – 190 – 210)
    (Cognitive-Theoretic Model of the Universe)

- Edith Stern (IQ score – 200+)
    (PhD Mathematics, engineer/inventor at IBM)

- Kim Ung-Yong (IQ score – 210)
    (PhD Civil Engineering, Researcher/Professor, South Korea)

- Christopher Hirata (IQ score – 225)
    PhD, professor, Ohio State University

- Terence Tao (IQ score – 225 – 230)
    co-recipient of Fields Medal, Nobel equivalent

---

[23] https://www.scienceabc.com › Humans.

The following information has been included to provide a reference point for the meaning of intelligence and its variables. The chart provides a concise analysis of the ranges of intellectual disability severity by IQ scores.[24]

Classifications of Intellectual Disability Severity

Severity Category	Approximate Percent Distribution of Cases by Severity	DSM-IV Criteria (severity levels were based only on IQ categories)	DSM-5 Criteria (severity classified on the basis of daily skills)	AAIDD Criteria (severity classified on the basis of intensity of support needed)	SSI Listings Criteria (The SSI listings do not specify severity levels, but indicate different standards for meeting or equaling listing level severity.)
Mild	85%	Approx. IQ range 50-69	Can live independently with minimum levels of support.	Intermittent support needed during transitions or periods of uncertainty.	IQ of 60 through 70 *and* a physical or other mental impairment imposing an additional and significant limitation of function
Moderate	10%	Approx. IQ range 36-49	Independent living may be achieved with moderate levels of support, such as those available in group homes.	Limited support needed in daily situations.	A valid verbal, performance, or full-scale IQ of 59 or less
Severe	3.5%	Approx. IQ range 20-35	Requires daily assistance with self-care activities and safety supervision.	Extensive support needed for daily activities.	A valid verbal, performance, or full-scale IQ of 59 or less
Profound	1.5%	IQ <20	Requires 24-hour care.	Pervasive support needed for every aspect of daily routines.	A valid verbal, performance, or full-scale IQ of 59 or less

---

[24] As set forth in the National Library of Medicine: https://www.ncbi.nlm.nih.gov/books/NBK332877/

No discussion about intelligence would be complete without a discussion of how some very intelligent people may have difficulty with the nuances of social interaction, appropriate behaviors, understanding social cues, and such. A classic example of this is Dr. Sheldon Cooper, a genius theoretical physicist, on the popular television sitcom, *The Big Bang Theory*. Dr. Cooper is clearly one of the brightest individuals on the show, yet he demonstrates narcissism, a lack of understanding of appropriate social interactions, an inability to perceive social cues, difficulty recognizing emotions, and obsessive-compulsive actions. His childlike behavior and intolerance of those with lesser abilities is extreme.

Despite that, he is a lovable character, expertly played by Jim Parsons. When the creators of *The Big Bang Theory* were asked if Sheldon was autistic, they said no, he was just "Sheldon." Despite his atypical personality he is a beloved character and watched by millions of people on this top-rated show.

All of us know someone who has a characteristic or two that may be similar to Sheldon's. They could be a quirky family member, a neighbor, or a coworker. We all have different strengths and weaknesses. Someone with a high IQ may not have any social awareness, they may appear as having an impairment. Recognizing that intelligence is manifested in many ways, we need to be tolerant. Indeed, the recognition and respect of individuals' differences makes us human. What is interesting is that *The Big Bang Theory* has helped to open a discussion about these issues. Just because someone is intelligent does not mean that they may not demonstrate inappropriate behaviors.

Responding to persons with intellectual disabilities. People with intellectual disabilities may have impairments in the areas listed below. The extent of the person's impairment determines the individual's limitations and the amount of assistance the individual may need. The level of support and assistance that would be required could be total care, moderate or minimal assistance.

For law enforcement officers, firefighters, EMTs, paramedics and other first responders, it is important to recognize that these individuals may have difficulties and limitations in the following areas:

- The activities of daily living and self-care, such as: bathing, dressing, eating, using the toilet, grooming, etc.

- Speech—may not be able to communicate;
  ~ Note that some people may communicate using a communication board that may have words or pictures, others may have a computerized communication device.

- Learning, reasoning and problem solving

- Understanding, signs, symbols, sounds, danger in general, danger from strangers, etc.

- The concept of time may be difficult for a person with this type of impairment. Therefore, asking the question of what time something happened may not work. Try to frame your question by putting it into a context that has meaning to them, such as: "was it before or after breakfast, lunch etc.?" "Were you watching TV?" "What show was on?" "Was it bedtime?" This provides a time frame that has meaning and relevance to the person, and may be the best approximation you will obtain.

How to respond:

- Approach the individual in a calm, nonthreatening manner.

- Do not get too close, give the person some space, don't touch the individual. You do not want to appear threatening.

- Introduce yourself and be respectful.

- If you are in a nosy area consider moving to a quieter one with less distractions.

- Recognize that the person may be frightened and or overwhelmed. They may be unable to determine if you are there to help or hurt them.

- Keep it simple, use concrete terms such as "show me," "tell me," "follow me," etc.

- Use appropriate language.

- Allow additional time for the individual to process information.

Just because the person may have difficulty with verbal communication does not mean that they do not understand. Individuals with intellectual disabilities may understand what you are saying—this is receptive language—but may not be able to verbally respond—this is expressive language. In this case, questions calling for "yes" and "no" answers would be best.

The individual may be able to indicate their response by shaking their head, or another method. You will need to try and determine what works. For example, ask the person, "How do you say 'yes'?" "How do you say, 'no'?" Examine the way in which they respond. Do they answer verbally? Do they shake their head? Do they move their body in a specific way? Do their eyes gaze to the left, right, up or down? Note their response so that you have a baseline, a consistent response for the simple yes or no answers.

Don't raise your voice or shout. This doesn't help, the issue is understanding not whether or not they hear you.

- Try to gather some identifying information from the individual.

- If possible, determine if the person has a caregiver or family member, and contact them.

- Do not discount what they have to say because of their disability. They may have pertinent information to offer.

- Monitor how you speak to the individual, don't talk down to the person.

- Speak directly to the individual, don't talk about them to others in front of them. This could be perceived as condescending and rude.

- Avoid sudden movements.

- Don't joke with the person, they may interpret it incorrectly.

- Determine if the person is injured. If that is the case, call an ambulance immediately. The individual may not be able to explain their injury and may be more seriously injured than what is apparent.

- Very serious consideration should be given to any situation that would require an arrest. Due to the person's disability, you may not have a satisfactory assessment of the person's physical condition. The individual may have a medical condition that is not obvious. Look for a medical alert ID, either around their wrist or neck.

- Since you are unaware of the person's medical condition, your best option may be to call for an ambulance.

- Recognize that making the decision to use medical transport provides the best chance for the safety of the person at the scene. Transporting the person in a patrol car or police van may be a bad idea.

Teenager with Intellectual Impairment Arrested for Drugs

Ty lived in a rough neighborhood in South Jersey. He liked to hang out with the older kids on the street after school. He was approached and asked to take a small paper bag across the street to the local bar. One of the cool guys gave him a few bucks and a candy bar. Ty was excited, he wanted the cool guys to like him. Ty took the bag across the street and was promptly arrested. The bar was being watched by police. Once in custody, it was obvious to the officers that Ty did not have any involvement in the drug ring. Ty was not upset; the officers gave him a soda and a bag of chips. Ty chattered about the event, and the officers paid attention.

At first, it didn't seem like Ty could identify the main drug dealer, but in Ty's chatter there began to emerge a few important details. Since Ty hung out on the street corner, he saw things that caught his attention. He said one of the guys would come around and stay in the playground across the street. Ty would see him at the playground. Ty said the man didn't like to play. He would just stand or sit. He would come with a kid sometimes; the kid would go on the swings. Ty referred to the man as "Rainbows." The officer asked Ty to describe what the man looked like. Ty wasn't sure, but he shared what he did know. Ty told the officers that "Rainbows" had "a stone in his nose." When asked if that was the man's name, Ty responded, "No, I made it up, because he had rainbow glasses." According to Ty, Rainbows would sit and watch the bar. Rainbows did not come every day. Ty did not know what day of the week Rainbows would come. But what he did know was that it happened on the "last day of school."

Upon further questioning, the officers were able to determine that the last day of school, was every Friday, before the weekend, and Ty didn't go to school on the weekends. According to Ty, "Rainbows, the big dealer man" would come and sit at the playground every Friday afternoon. When asked about what time he would come, Ty responded just before I eat dinner, when it turns dark. The officers had not been successful in apprehending the major drug dealer. But Ty and seen him many times. The officers continued to question Ty. Although he was not able to answer the questions in a typical manner, the perceptive officers continued to chat with him and Ty continued talking. He was able to describe the dealer but not in the usual way. Ultimately, the officers located and arrested "Rainbows."

> Sure enough, "Rainbows" had fancy glasses with colorful side pieces, and "Rainbows" did have a shiny stone in his nose, his nose was pierced, and there was a shiny stone in the piercing. "Rainbows" was there in the late afternoon on a Friday, when it began to get dark, just about the time Ty had dinner.
>
> This is a true story told to me when I was a school principal. Ty attended our school, and Ty's mom told me of his adventure; clearly, she was relieved that everything had turned out OK and that Ty was safe. In this instance Ty was in the wrong place at the wrong time. He was asked to do something illegal but had no idea that what he was doing was unlawful; he simply did not perceive it as wrong. It was obvious that the people in the neighborhood knew that Ty had an intellectual impairment and used him to carry drugs. Who knows how many times this may have happened. This could have gone terribly wrong. Teenagers with intellectual disabilities are extraordinarily vulnerable and easily victimized.
>
> The officers in this case were patient and perceptive. They realized Ty was not knowingly and willfully committing a crime but being used. They carefully listened to what Ty had to say and realized that his information could help identify a suspect. Although Ty did not present the information in the usual way, he was able to relay important and relevant information that led to an arrest. The officers were rewarded for the patience, in listening to this teenager's explanation, they discovered the information they needed. Ty cooperated in the only way he knew how.

When interviewing a person with special needs, be patient. Just because they may not be able to answer your questions in a typical manner, does not mean that they don't have relevant facts.

- If an incident is reported by a teen with special needs, pay close attention.

- The incident may be interpreted differently, but the events may have actually taken place.

Response & Assessment – Part II

- Do not discard information from a person with a disability, there may be enough facts presented to determine what actually happened.

- Listen to their retelling of events, there may be just enough truth and evidence provided, such as a "hidden clue."

- Even if an event appears farfetched, they are seeing it from a different perspective; their information may help your case, do not discard their story. There just may be enough facts and details in their story that may seem insignificant at the time but will prove to be relevant and important later. Let them talk and carefully document the details in your report.

Bullets as Toys

The police arrived at the school at 9:30 am, and asked to see the principal. They were called by a bus driver who reported that a student had bullets on the bus. The student was observed by the bus driver and bus aide holding the bullets. The police, who were very familiar with the school and knew that the school served special needs students, arrived immediately. The social worker and the principal were both present during the questioning because the student, Tyrell, was only 12 years old. When Tyrell was asked if he had bullets, he was confused. He scratched his head and said what? The officers explained what a bullet looked like. Tyrell answered, "Oh, you mean these?" Tyrell pulled 4 bullets from his pocket. He put them on the table and said, "These are my friends, I found them on my street." He pointed to the first bullet and said, "This is Earl, this is Sam, this is J, and this is T. We play together and I like them."

Tyrell lived in a very tough, crime-ridden neighborhood. He had no concept of danger, did not understand what a bullet was, and thought they were objects he could play with. The officers took possession of the bullets, and they and the principal contacted Tyrell's parent to inform her what had

> occurred. Tyrell was not arrested. The officers contacted the police department in Tyrell's city and informed them that bullets were found in the area around the student's home. The incident was documented and properly handled. Since the police knew the type of students the school served, they were well informed of the protocol for the students and the unique challenges they faced.

The takeaway: The situation is not always as it appears on the surface. A report of bullets and kids presents a frightening image. It calls for immediate attention. The bus driver and aide were right in contacting the police. The officers handled the situation well because of their training, experience and prior knowledge of the students attending the school.

§6.3. Multiple Disabilities

A person with *multiple disabilities* has more than one disabling condition. The impairment substantially limits major life activities. The person could be in a wheelchair, have a speech impairment as well as health issues. An individual may have two, three or more conditions. Since this term covers many variables, it describes the most severe type of disability that impacts the individual's ability to carry out activities of daily living without some type of assistance. The severity of the person's limitations determines the level of impairment, which may be moderate to severe or profound.

It is important to keep in mind that a person may become seriously disabled later in life. Circumstances such as a car accident, a fall, a stroke, surgery or other medical conditions such as multiple sclerosis (MS) or amyotrophic lateral sclerosis (ALS), commonly known as Lou Gehrig's disease, can occur in mid-life. People who have these illnesses may be affected physically, but their mental capacity may be intact. Therefore, do not assume that someone with a severe physical disability has an intellectual impairment.

Response & Assessment – Part II

A person with multiple disabilities may have:

- limited mobility, difficulty walking, need a cane or a walker, or be in a wheelchair

- limited use of their hands, arms or legs

- an inability to move (paralysis)

- slurred or limited speech, no speech, or use a communication device

- mild or moderate vision loss, or blindness

- perceptual limitations, which limits their ability to understand what they see

- mild or moderate hearing loss, or deafness

- significant health issues

- difficulty breathing

- difficulty swallowing

- twitching or spasms

- difficulty processing information, or may not understand what is being said, or unable to understand the meaning of the information provided

- an inability to move independently without assistance

- the need for assistance with all activities of daily living and self-care, such as bathing, dressing, using the toilet, eating, and mobility

- mild, moderate or severe cognitive impairment

- the need to utilize a service animal (which is protected under the Americans with Disabilities Act and Section 504 of the Rehabilitation Act of 1973)

How to Respond

- Approach the individual in a calm, nonthreatening manner.

- Do not get too close, give the person some space, don't touch the individual.

- Do not touch or lean on the person's wheelchair or walker, this is just like touching the person, it is seen as invading their personal space.

- Introduce yourself and be respectful.

- Do not assume that the person is unable to understand or communicate; however, you will be able to determine this quickly.

- Create a safe atmosphere, if possible, if you are in a noisy area, consider moving to a quieter one with fewer distractions.

- Don't raise your voice or shout; this doesn't help. The issue is understanding, not whether or not they hear you.

- Recognize that the person may be frightened and/or overwhelmed.

- Allow adequate time for your interview.

- If there is a caretaker or family member nearby ask them for assistance, *if appropriate*.
    ~ In the circumstance of an accident, this would be important. In a domestic violence situation, you may have to separate family members to determine what is happening. The person with the disability may be the victim here, and afraid to communicate in front of the

caretaker or family member. This situation is dicey, i.e., a family member, service provider or caretaker may want to protect themselves or the offender. They may not provide truthful information.

- Speak directly to the person, keep it simple. Do not talk too much. Ask your question and stop; wait for the answer.
    ~ This is critical. It is at this point that you will determine if they can respond. If the person does not respond, ask again, and wait. This is when you will know if the person can communicate.
    ~ As with persons with intellectual disabilities, just because the person may have difficulty with verbal communication does not mean that they do not understand. The person may understand what you are saying—this is receptive language—but may not be able to verbally respond—this is expressive language. In this case, questions calling for "yes" and "no" answers would be best.
    ~ The individual may be able to indicate their response by shaking their head, or another method. You will need to try and determine what works. For example, ask the person, "How do you say 'yes'?" "How do you say, 'no'?" Examine the way in which they respond. Do they answer verbally? Do they shake their head? Do they move their body in a specific way? Do their eyes gaze to the left, right, up or down? Note their response so that you can have a baseline, which is a consistent response for simple "yes" or "no" questions.

- If the person is in a facility, such has an assisted living center, an adult day care unit, or nursing home, it is critical to speak to the person with the assistance of the facility social worker. If the person is reporting abuse, or violence in the facility, it may be necessary to call an outside agency to assist in your interview.

- Try to gather some identifying information from the individual.

- Help the person by asking specific questions.
  - ~ Don't say, "Tell me what happened." First try to pinpoint a time frame. Ask, "When did it happen? Before breakfast? After lunch?" This way the person has to indicate in only a few words. Try to identify a time frame since the individual may not be able to state a precise time. Their day may be divided into routine times, use their schedule as a reference point to determine the time of day. If the person answers "snack time," you may find out that snack time is at 2:30 in the afternoon every day.
  - ~ The person may say, "It happened after *Wheel of Fortune*." This is important information. The individual was not able give you a precise time, but the time can be determined by finding out what time *Wheel of Fortune* is aired.

- Ask simple direct questions, don't ask anything requiring speculation or abstract thought, such as, "Why would she do that?" or "Where do you think they went?"

- Examples of effective questions:
  - ~ "Was it a man or a woman?'
  - ~ "What color was the person's hair?" If the person cannot say a color point to something in the room, ask, "Was it this color?"
  - ~ "Do you know the person?"
  - ~ "What is their name?"
  - ~ "Did he or she hit you?" "Show me where."
  - ~ "Did you fall down?"

This is a slow process and takes some time. Don't dismiss the information the individual is providing. They may have witnessed a crime, seen someone steal, witnessed abuse or violence in a facility, or may be a victim of abuse or violence in a facility or in their home. They may have been in an accident or been hurt. It is easy to lose patience and become frustrated when information is so difficult to obtain. Remember that this person is frustrated too; she wants to tell you what happened and she is upset.

Response & Assessment – Part II

If the incident is an accident, you may not be able to determine if the person is injured or the extent of the injuries. The best and safest decision is to always call an ambulance immediately. Time is of the essence. The individual may not be able to explain what happened or be able to describe the extent of his or her injury or be aware of any injury; they may be more seriously injured than what is apparent.

> **February, 2018 – I Need Lipstick!**
>
> A police officer responded to a call to assist on an ambulance run from a nursing home. An elderly woman with multiple disabilities needed to be transported to the local hospital. The ambulance was already at the scene when the young police officer arrived. The woman was very agitated and fearful. She was yelling that she didn't want to go to the hospital, and was giving the nurses and paramedics a hard time. The officer went into the room and began to speak with the woman. The officer was trying to get the woman to calm down.
>
> He began to tell the woman how pretty she was and began to actually flirt with this nursing home resident. He said he was sure that if she wasn't going to the hospital he would ask her on a date, and she could have dinner with him. The woman began to respond in a positive way. She stopped yelling and calmed down and actually began to flirt back! She told the officer that he was handsome, and she would love to have dinner with him. She said, "I'll be back dear," and "I'll go out to dinner with you then!" The situation calmed down significantly and the officer said goodbye and left. As the paramedics were wheeling the woman down the corridor she started to yell, "I have nothing to wear! I have to get my hair done, and I need lipstick!" The woman started to get agitated all over again. She believed the officer was serious; she could not distinguish between reality and fantasy.
>
> This was a true event. It was reported by someone visiting their parent at that nursing home and was reported

> to this author. The officer did help the woman calm down; however, his method was inappropriate and ill advised. He was trying to be helpful but did not realize that the woman could not make the distinction between joking and reality.

§6.4. Orthopedic Impairment

Orthopedic impairments include a wide variety of disorders that may adversely affect a person's activities of daily living and/or physical performance. There are three categories of orthopedic impairment: neuromotor impairments, degenerative diseases and musculoskeletal disorders. The severity of the condition depends on many factors and may be mild, moderate or severe to profound. No two individuals are the same. In fact, two individuals may have the exact same diagnosis, yet their capabilities may be different.

A neuromotor impairment is an abnormality of, or damage to, the brain, the spinal cord or the nervous system. It can occur prenatal, before birth, or during birth. Examples of the most common neuromotor impairments are: cerebral palsy, seizure disorders (epilepsy) and spina bifida.

Cerebral palsy is characterized by abnormal, involuntary and/or uncoordinated movements, which may or may not affect intellectual functioning. People with the disease may have difficulty speaking. To assist the person, there are a variety of communication devices, from the simplest language board to a sophisticated electronic communication system. Cerebral palsy can affect either the arms or legs, or both the arms and legs. It can also be found on only one side of the body, which is called hemiplegia (on the left or right side).

The term paraplegia refers to the involvement of only the legs, while the term quadriplegia refers to the involvement of all four limbs.[25] As with other conditions, it may be mild, moderate or severe to profound. A person with a mild case could be able to walk, talk, work, drive and live their life with minor adaptations. A person with

---

[25] http://www.projectidealonline.org/v/orthopedic-impairments/

a moderate form of cerebral palsy could use a wheelchair, either motorized or self-propelled, and function generally well with moderate assistance for some self-care needs. A person with severe involvement would need extensive support for all activities of daily living.

Spina bifida is a congenital birth defect, where the spinal column does not close all the way. The actual meaning of the words spina bifida means split-spine. As with other conditions, it can range from mild to severe to profound. Spina bifida can result in some paralysis. Intellectual functioning may or may not be affected. Some people with the condition may have difficulty walking, some may require a wheelchair and have problems with bowel or bladder control.

Degenerative diseases are a type of medical condition. There are various diseases in this category that cause tissues and organs of your body to change over time. Some degenerative diseases do not show up until later in life, such as Parkinson's and osteoarthritis, whereas muscular dystrophy affects children.

Musculoskeletal disorders are disorders that affect the movement of the human body's musculoskeletal system, including muscles, tendons, ligaments, nerves, discs, blood vessels, etc. The disability can range from a limb amputation, fractures, joint or spine conditions, club foot, dwarfism, rheumatoid arthritis, paralysis, soft tissue injury (burns) as well as the many other specific conditions identified by the Social Security Administration.

Characteristics of individuals with these conditions. These persons:

- may be in a wheelchair
- may use canes, walkers, or crutches
- may have difficulty with balance
- may have an assistive communication device for speech
- may have slurred speech
- may have a service animal
- may have difficulty with gross and fine motor skills

- may require assistance with activities of daily living and self-care, such as bathing, dressing, using the toilet, eating, and mobility
- may have average, limited or impaired intellectual functioning
- may have other medical conditions not apparent (such as a seizure disorder)
- may have limited use of their hands, arms, legs
- may have very tight muscles (spastic)
- may have difficulty with balance and have involuntary movements
- may have limited ability to move (paralysis)
- may have difficulty with writing, reading, and problem solving
- may have poor muscle control and coordination
- may drool
- may have hearing loss
- may grind their teeth
- may have a physical deformity

How to Respond

- Approach the individual in a calm, nonthreatening manner.
- Do not get too close, give the person some space, don't touch the individual.
- Do not touch or lean on the person's wheelchair or walker, this is just like touching the person, it is seen as invading their personal space.
- Introduce yourself and be respectful.
- Do not assume that the person is unable to understand or communicate; you will be able to determine this quickly.

- Create a safe atmosphere, if possible; if you are in a noisy area, consider moving to a quieter one with fewer distractions.

- Don't raise your voice or shout; this doesn't help. The issue is understanding, not whether or not they hear you.

- Recognize that the person may be frightened and/or overwhelmed.

- Allow adequate time for your interview.

- If there is a caretaker or family member nearby ask them for assistance, if appropriate.
    - ~ In the circumstance of an accident, this would be important. In a domestic violence situation, you may have to separate family members to determine what is happening. The person with the disability may be the victim here, and afraid to communicate in front of the caretaker or family member. This situation is dicey, i.e., a family member, service provider or caretaker may want to protect themselves or the offender. They may not provide truthful information.

- If the person is in a facility, such as an assisted-living center, an adult day care unit, or nursing home, it is critical to speak to the person with the assistance of the facility social worker. If the person is reporting abuse, or violence in the facility, it may be necessary to call an outside agency to assist in your interview. Depending on the outcome of the interview, you may need to report the facility to the state agency that monitors nursing homes.

- Speak directly to the person and keep it simple. Do not talk too much. Ask your question and stop; wait for the answer.
    - ~ This is critical. It is at this point that you will determine if they can respond. If the person does not respond, ask again, and wait. This is when you will know if the person can communicate.
    - ~ As with persons with intellectual disabilities, just because the person may have difficulty with verbal communi-

cation does not mean that they do not understand. The person may understand what you are saying—this is *receptive* language—but may not be able to verbally respond—this is *expressive* language. In this case, questions calling for "yes" and "no" answers would be best.

~ The individual may be able to indicate their response by shaking their head, or another method. You will need to try and determine what works. For example, ask the person, "How do you say 'yes'?" "How do you say, 'no'?" Examine the way in which they respond. Do they answer verbally? Do they shake their head? Do they move their body in a specific way? Do their eyes gaze to the left, right, up or down? Note their response so that you can have a baseline, a consistent response for the simple "yes" or "no" questions.

- Try to gather some identifying information from the individual.

- Help the person by asking specific questions.
    ~ Don't say, "Tell me what happened." First try to pinpoint a time frame. Ask, "When did it happen? Before breakfast? After lunch?" This way the person has to indicate in only a few words. Try to identify a time frame since the individual may not be able to state a precise time. Their day may be divided into routine times, use their schedule as a reference point to determine the time of day. If the person answers "snack time," you may find out that snack time is at 2:30 in the afternoon every day.
    ~ The person may say, it happened after a particular television show. This is important information. The individual was not able give you a precise time, but the time can be determined by finding out what time that show is aired.

- Ask simple direct questions, don't ask anything requiring speculation or abstract thought, such as, "Why would she do that?" or "Where do you think they went?"

- Examples of effective questions:
  - "Was it a man or a woman?'
  - "What color was the person's hair?" If the person cannot say a color point to something in the room, ask, "Was it this color?"
  - "Do you know the person?"
  - "What is their name?"
  - "Did he/she hit you?" "Show me where."
  - "Did you fall down?"

This is a slow process and takes some time. Don't dismiss the information the individual is providing. They may have witnessed a crime, seen someone steal, witnessed abuse or violence in a facility, or may be a victim of abuse or violence in a facility or in their home. They may have been in an accident or been hurt. It is easy to lose patience and become frustrated when information is so difficult to obtain. Remember that this person is frustrated too; she wants to tell you what happened and she is upset.

If the incident is an accident, you may not be able to determine if the person is injured or the extent of the injuries. The best and safest decision is to always call an ambulance immediately. Time is of the essence. The individual may not be able to explain what happened or be able to describe the extent of his or her injury or be aware of any injury; they may be more seriously injured than what is apparent.

Burglary Gone Wrong!

The idea was a simple one—Get their friend Ray to assist in a burglary. Ray's job would be to climb into the air shaft of the building. Ray would open the vent above the store, throw a rope down to the floor, and use the rope to propel himself down. Ray would then use his arms to "walk" over to the door, open it, and let the other guys in. They would rob the store and carry Ray out. Ray was paralyzed from the waist down, but had tremendous upper-body strength. Ray could balance himself on his hands and arms and support his body weight by his arms. He was also a small and agile guy, who could easily maneuver in a small space. Ray left his wheelchair in the side alley, got into the building, as planned, and into the store.

The plan seemed to work until the store alarm was triggered. Ray's friends ran and left him there. When the police arrived at the scene, Ray was found in the store sitting on the floor, weaponless and distraught. Being very resourceful, he cried out, "*My Legs! My Legs! I can't move my legs! My friends threw me down from the ceiling and now I can't move my legs! They left me here, I need a doctor!*" Ray wailed on and on, "*The Pain, oh the Pain!*" "*They made me do it and left me!*" "*Now I'm a cripple!*" Ray really hammed it up. The officers immediately called for an ambulance and Ray was accompanied to the hospital by an officer. When the remaining officers found the wheelchair in the alley, they knew that Ray had pulled a fast one. This is a true event. I knew Ray, he had been a student of mine. When the story hit the local newspaper, I was shocked. In this incident, Ray demonstrated his resourcefulness, using his disability to his advantage. Subsequently, Ray was put on probation for his part in the robbery.

The takeaway: Just like those without disabilities, a person with a disability or impairment could be involved in illegal activities.

§6.5. Other Health Impaired

The term "other health impaired" refers to persons having limited strength, vitality, or alertness, including a heightened alertness to environmental stimuli, that results in limited alertness with respect to the person's surrounding environment.

This condition may be due to:

- chronic or acute health problems such as asthma
- attention deficit disorder, or attention deficit hyperactivity disorder
- diabetes
- epilepsy
- heart conditions
- hemophilia
- lead poisoning
- leukemia
- nephritis (a kidney disorder) or rheumatic fever
- sickle cell anemia
- Tourette syndrome

§6.6. Specific Learning Disabilities

A "specific learning disability" means a disorder in one or more of the basic psychological processes involved in understanding or in using language, spoken or written. The disability may manifest itself by the individual having difficulties with abilities to listen, think, speak, read, write, spell, or to do mathematical calculations, including conditions such as perceptual disabilities, brain injury, minimal brain dysfunction, dyslexia, and developmental aphasia. Learning disabilities effect how a person functions in their environment and can have a significant impact on their life.

> **"I was giving the gun a ride"**
>
> On a Saturday night in southern New Jersey, a car was stopped for speeding. As the officer approached the vehicle, he observed a gun in plain view on the back seat of the vehicle. The officer calls for backup. The person driving the car is a 19-year-old male who states, "I'm special ed." The driver is asked to get out of the car and is handcuffed. He repeatedly states, "I'm special ed." When he is asked about the gun he responded, "I was giving it a ride." The driver was cooperative and was arrested without incident. It was later determined that the driver was a telling the truth, he was a special education student. But the fact that he had a disability did not excuse him from the crime of unlawful possession of a handgun.

The takeaway: Having a disability does not exempt someone from the law.

The subcategories of Specific Learning Disabilities and their characteristics include:

Auditory Processing Disorders:

- The person has difficulty understanding spoken language.
- The person hears what is said but cannot process the information.
- The person has difficulty understanding and following verbal directions.
- The person is easily distracted by noise.

Aphasia:

- This condition affects speech and language.
- The person has difficulty speaking or comprehending speech.
- The person has difficulty with reading and listening.
- The person has difficulty with word retrieval, can't think of the right word.

~ People who have had a stroke struggle with aphasia. They may have difficulty remembering the names of objects and also struggle with word usage and the flow of speech.

Dyscalculia:

- The person has difficulty with mathematics.
- The person has difficulty grasping calculations, math processes and their applications.

Dysgraphia:

- The person has difficulty with handwriting.
- The person may experience problems with holding a pencil, writing letters in words of unequal size, and spacing issues.

Dyslexia:

- A very common learning disability that involves difficulty learning to identify letters, learning to spell, and read and write.
- Once the individual learns to write, words may be misspelled, letters and numbers may be transposed, reversed, omitted and repeated.
- The person may have excellent listening skills and may be bright and articulate.

Dyspraxia:

- A developmental disability that affects coordination.
- The person has difficulty with fine and or gross motor coordination.
- The person may have issues with walking, balance and hand dexterity.
- The condition may also affect speech.

Sensory Processing Disorder:

- A neurological disorder originally called Sensory Integration Dysfunction.
- With this condition, the brain has difficulty receiving and responding to information that comes from one or more of the five senses.
- The person may be overly sensitive to loud sounds, bright or flashing lights.
- The person may be overly sensitive to touch, texture and taste.
- The person may be hypersensitve to the feel of some clothes, or shoes, etc.
- The person may be overly sensitive to the feel, the look, and/or the taste of food.

Visual Processing Disorder:

- This disorder causes difficulty in the way the brain processes and interprets visual information and makes sense of information seen through the eyes.
- The individual may have perfect vision; this is not a sight issue.
- The eye may see a triangle, but the brain may interpret it as a square.
- Individuals may have a hard time recognizing the difference between objects, and learning letters and numbers.
- The person may have difficulty learning to read.

§6.7. Traumatic Brain Injury

Traumatic brain injury (TBI) happens when a bump, blow, jolt, or other head injury causes damage to the brain. Every year, millions of people in the United States suffer brain injuries. More than half are bad enough that people must go to the hospital. The worst

Response & Assessment – Part II

injuries can lead to permanent brain damage or death.[26] This may occur as a result of a car accident, a blow to the head, a sports injury, or a fall.

Characteristics:[27]

Moderate to severe traumatic brain injuries can include any of the signs and symptoms of mild injury, as well as these symptoms that may appear within the first hours to days after a head injury:

- may have immediate or delayed symptoms
- may have a concussion, nausea, vomiting, drowsiness
- blurry vision
- headaches
- slurred speech
- confusion, from moderate to profound
- irritability
- agitation, combativeness or other unusual behavior
- loss of consciousness, for a minute or a few minutes, or longer
- dazed; dizziness; loss of balance
- ringing in the ears
- sensitive to light and/or sound
- memory and concentration problems
- may have convulsions or seizures
- dilation of pupils in one or both eyes
- fluids draining from the nose or ears
- weakness or numbness in fingers and or toes
- loss of coordination
- convulsions or seizures
- bad taste in the mouth or changes in the ability to smell

---

[26] https://medlineplus.gov/traumaticbraininjury.html.
[27] https://www.mayoclinic.org/diseases-conditions/traumatic-brain-injury/symptoms-causes/syc-20378557.

How to Respond:

If you are responding to a scene, whether a crime scene, a domestic dispute, a car accident, or another event and observe any of the signs characterized above,

- *immediately call for an ambulance to have the individual transported to the nearest hospital.*
- *it is essential that you seek emergency medical care for an individual if there are any signs or symptoms of traumatic brain injury following a recent blow or other traumatic injury to the head.*[28]

The terms "mild," "moderate" and "severe" are used to describe the effect of the injury on brain function. A mild injury to the brain is still a serious injury that requires prompt attention and an accurate diagnosis.[29]

§6.8. Breathing Issues

If someone says they are having problems breathing, BELIEVE THEM! **Just because a person can speak does not mean that they will be able to continue to speak.** This is not an accurate assessment of the ability to breathe. The feeling of not being able to breathe quickly worsens. According to the Mayo Clinic, most cases of shortness of breath are due to heart or lung conditions. If a person suddenly has shortness of breath it can be a serious medical emergency, and should not be ignored. The best course of action is to get immediate medical attention.

It may be from any of these causes:

- Asthma (bronchospasm)
- Carbon monoxide poisoning

---

[28] https://www.mayoclinic.org/diseases-conditions/traumatic-brain-injury/symptoms-causes/syc-20378557.

[29] *Id.*

- Cardiac tamponade (excess fluid around the heart)
- Heart attack
- Heart failure
- Low blood pressure (hypotension)
- Pneumonia (and other pulmonary infections)
- Pneumothorax (collapsed lung)
- Pulmonary embolism (blood clot in an artery in the lung)
- Sudden blood loss
- Broken ribs
- Swelling of the lid of your windpipe
- Inhalation of a foreign object, choking on food, candy, etc.
- Upper airway obstruction (blockage in the breathing passage) [30]

Pleading suspect dies in police custody:

From the moment the Los Angeles police handcuffed him, Jorge Azucena told officers he needed help. "I can't breathe, I can't breathe," he pleaded. "I have asthma, I have asthma." It was reported that many officers heard the suspect's request for medical attention, but did nothing. "You can breathe just fine," one sergeant told him. "You can talk, so you can breathe." [31]

By the time the suspect was booked, he could not walk or stand. He repeatedly said he had asthma and could not breathe. He was carried into a cell and quickly became unconscious. When the paramedics arrived, he was dead.

"There should not be any question that when somebody in custody is heard to say 'I cannot breathe,' the officers should promptly call for an ambulance," said Robert Saltzman, a member of the Police Commission that oversees the LAPD. [32]

---

[30] https://www.mayoclinic.org/symptoms/shortness-of-breath/basics/causes/sym-20050890.
[31] http://www.latimes.com/local/crime/la-me-lapd-custody-death-20140823-story.html.
[32] *Id.*

If you have a suspect on the ground and are kneeling down on them, you may be interfering with their breathing. If you have them handcuffed, chest down on the ground, and are using your body weight to hold them down, you may be interfering with their ability to breathe. If the person has asthma, their airway could be compromised very quickly.

As a rule of thumb: **ALWAYS BELIEVE A PERSON WHEN THEY TELL YOU THEY CANNOT BREATHE.**

> *On July 17, 2014, Eric Garner died in Staten Island, New York City, after a New York City Police Department (NYPD) officer put him in a headlock for about 15 to 19 seconds while arresting him. NYPD policy prohibits the use of chokeholds. The officer denied choking Garner, but the New York City Medical Examiner's Office report stated "Cause of Death: Compression of neck, compression of chest and prone positioning during physical restraint by police" and "Contributing Conditions: 'Acute and chronic bronchial asthma; Obesity; Hypertensive cardiovascular disease.'" Garner was heard eleven times saying I can't breathe while lying face down on the sidewalk.*[33]

---

[33] https://en.wikipedia.org/wiki/Death_of_Eric_Garner

KEY POINTS

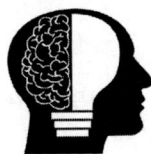

- Recent statistics show that about 1 in 5 Americans have a mental illness.

- Suicide, is the tenth leading cause of death in the United States and the second leading cause of death among people aged 19 to 34.

- By itself, mental illness does not predict violence, but having a mental illness and a substance abuse problem does increase the risk of violence.

- A dangerous situation can occur when individuals with mental illnesses may provoke police into killing them. This is now commonly known as "Suicide by Cop" (SBC).

- When a mentally ill person decides to initiate a "Suicide by Cop" incident, they generally have a premeditated, well-thought out plan.

- People who engage in "Suicide by Cop" may choose this method to avoid the shameful consequences of killing oneself, to avoid the exclusions from life insurance policies so that their families may collect the benefits, and may rationalize that it avoids the religious and spiritual tenets against suicide, thereby saving face.

- People who engage in "Suicide by Cop" may choose this method to communicate hopelessness, depression, or desperation.

KEY POINTS (Continued)

- Characteristics of mental illness include: inappropriate responses; talking but making no sense; hallucinations, hearing voices; delusions, paranoia; anxiety, panic, fright; an inability to make eye contact; and suicidal thoughts.

- A person with an *intellectual disability* has sub-average general intellectual functioning, along with deficits in both cognitive capacity and adaptive behavior.

- Intellectual disabilities are characterized by limitations in reasoning, learning, problem solving and adaptive behavior.

- An intellectual disability is not the same as a developmental disability.

- A person's Intelligence Quotient—one's IQ—is a statistical score determined by standardized tests used to measure human intelligence.

- There are multiple IQ tests comprised of questions in the areas of verbal and performance that measure general knowledge, language, reasoning, memory skills, conceptual skills, spatial, sequencing and problem-solving skills.

- Two types of intelligence that cannot be measured in the standard IQ test are: "Emotional Intelligence" (EQ) and "Social Intelligence" (SQ).

- Social Intelligence is more commonly referred to as tact, common sense, or street smarts.

- Emotional Intelligence is having "the ability to identify and manage your own emotions and the emotions of others."

KEY POINTS (Continued)

- Persons with profound intellectual disabilities may have difficulties and limitations in the activities of daily living and self-care, such as: bathing, dressing, eating, using the toilet, grooming, and speech.

- Persons with intellectual disabilities may understand what you are saying — this is *receptive* language — but may not be able to verbally respond — this is *expressive* language.

- A person with *multiple disabilities* has more than one disabling condition. The person could be in a wheelchair, have a speech impairment as well as health issues.

- There are three categories of orthopedic impairment; neuromotor impairments, degenerative diseases and musculoskeletal disorders.

- A neuromotor impairment is an abnormality of, or damage to, the brain, the spinal cord or the nervous system. It can occur prenatal, before birth, or during birth. Examples of the most common neuromotor impairments are: cerebral palsy, seizure disorders (epilepsy) and spinal bifida.

- The term paraplegia refers to the involvement of only the legs, whereas the term quadriplegia refers to the involvement of all four limbs.

- Musculoskeletal disorders are disorders that affect the movement of the human body's musculoskeletal system, including muscles, tendons, ligaments, nerves, discs, blood vessels, etc.

- The term "other health impaired" suggests the person may have, for example: chronic or acute health problems such as asthma; attention deficit disorder, or attention deficit hyperactivity disorder; diabetes; epilepsy; heart conditions; hemophilia; or Tourette syndrome.

KEY POINTS (Continued)

- A "specific learning disability" means a disorder in one or more of the basic psychological processes involved in understanding or in using language, spoken or written.

- Several examples of specific learning disabilities include: auditory processing disorders; aphasia; dyscalculia; dysgraphia; dyslexia; dyspraxia; and sensory or visual processing disorders.

- Traumatic brain injury victims may have or experience, a concussion, nausea, vomiting, drowsiness, blurry vision, headaches, slurred speech, confusion, loss of consciousness, dizziness, loss of balance. ringing in the ears, or seizures. They need immediate medical attention.

- If an officer has a suspect on the ground and is kneeling down on them, the officer may be interfering with the person's breathing. If the officer has the person handcuffed, chest down on the ground, and is using his body weight to hold the person down, the officer may be interfering with the person's ability to breathe.

- Always believe a person when they tell you they can't breathe. They need immediate medical assistance.

Chapter Seven
ADMISSIONS AND CONFESSIONS

§7.1. Introduction

The determination of an intellectual or cognitive impairment is not always simple, it can be a difficult process, even for a professional. Many times, however, the determination is easy because it is very obvious that the individual has some type of impairment. Yet there are times when this determination is as clear as mud. Essential to this discussion are the actions, demeanor and general conduct of the individual in question. Ask yourself these questions: Did the person appear oriented to time and space? Did the person appear to understand what was happening? Did you, as a public official, at any time question the person's cognitive capacity? Did you observe any unusual behavior or response that led you to believe that the individual had an intellectual impairment? Did the person respond appropriately because they understood what was occurring? The law provides some help in these cases. The courts have determined that if a reasonable person believes that the conduct of the individual appeared to be appropriate for the circumstances, the assumption that the individual is not impaired may be acceptable. If, at a later time, it is determined that the person has or had an intellectual impairment that was not apparent at the time of the arrest, the person's admission or confession may still be considered valid and admissible, particularly when the law enforcement official did not observe any behavior which indicated an impairment.

Properly secured admissions and confessions are integral in the law enforcement scheme and are extremely persuasive at trial. The ability to obtain a valid confession has been described as "not an evil but an unmitigated good."[1] As the United States Supreme Court observed in *McNeil v. Wisconsin*, "[a]dmissions of guilt resulting

---
[1] *McNeil v. Wisconsin*, 501 U.S. 171, 111 S. Ct. 2204, 2210 (1991).

from valid *Miranda* waivers are more than merely desirable; they are essential to society's compelling interest in finding, convicting, and punishing those who violate the law."[2] The introduction of an admission or a confession at trial "is like no other evidence. Indeed, 'the defendant's own confession is probably the most probative and damaging evidence that can be admitted against him. ... The admissions of a defendant come from the actor himself, the most knowledgeable and unimpeachable source of information about his past conduct. Certainly, confessions have profound impact on the jury[.]'"[3]

§7.2. The *Miranda* Rights

In *Miranda v. Arizona*,[4] the United States Supreme Court addressed "the admissibility of statements obtained from an individual who is subjected to custodial police interrogation and the necessity for procedures which assure that the individual is accorded his privilege under the Fifth Amendment to the Constitution not to be compelled to incriminate himself."[5] The Court ruled that "the privilege is fulfilled only when the person is guaranteed the right 'to remain silent unless he chooses to speak in the unfettered exercise of his own free will.'"[6]

"Coercive" custodial interrogation is the "evil" that the Court addressed in *Miranda*. "Custodial interrogation" is defined as "questioning initiated by law enforcement officers after a person has been taken into custody or otherwise deprived of his freedom of action in any significant way."[7] This concept of custodial interro-

---

[2] *Id.* 501 U.S. 171, 111 S. Ct. at 2210 (citation and internal quotes omitted).
[3] *Arizona v. Fulminante*, 499 U.S. 279, 296, 111 S. Ct. 1246, 1257 (1991) (quoting *Bruton v. United States*, 391 U.S. 123, 139-40, 88 S. Ct. 1620, 1630 (1968) (White, J., dissenting).
[4] *Miranda v. Arizona*, 384 U.S. 436, 86 S. Ct. 1602 (1966).
[5] *Miranda* at 439, 86 S. Ct. at 1609.
[6] *Id*, at 460, 86 S. Ct. at 1620 (quoting *Malloy v. Hogan*, 378 U.S. 1, 8, 84 S. Ct. 1489, 1493 (1964)).
[7] *Miranda v. Arizona*, 384 U.S. 436, 444, 86 S. Ct. 1602, 1612 (1966).

gation is what the Court had in mind when it previously "spoke of an investigation which had focused on an accused."[8]

The all-familiar requirements flowing from *Miranda* are as follows. Prior to custodial interrogation, the person must be informed:

- *You have the right to remain silent.*
- *Anything you say can and will be used against you in a court of law.*
- *You have the right to consult with an attorney and have an attorney present during questioning.*
- *If you cannot afford an attorney, one can be provided to you before questioning at no cost.*
- *You may ask for an attorney at any time during questioning, and questioning will stop if at any time you ask for an attorney.*

Thereafter, if the individual

indicates in any manner and at any stage of the process that he wishes to consult with an attorney before speaking there can be no questioning. Likewise, if the individual is alone and *indicates in any manner* that he does not wish to be interrogated, the police may not question him. The mere fact that he might have answered some questions on his own does not deprive him of the right to refrain from answering any further inquiries until he has consulted with an attorney and thereafter consents to be questioned.[9]

At court, the prosecution must demonstrate that the *Miranda* warnings were administered to the accused prior to any custodial interrogation. As emphasized in *Dickerson v. United States*,[10] the *Miranda* decision "laid down 'concrete constitutional guidelines for law

---

[8] *Id.* at 444 n.4, 86 S. Ct. at 1612 n.4 (1966) (referring to *Escobedo v. Illinois*, 378 U.S. 478, 84 S. Ct. 1758 (1964)).

[9] *Miranda v. Arizona*, 384 U.S. 436, 444-45, 86 S. Ct. 1602, 1612 (1966) (emphasis added).

[10] *Dickerson v. United States*, 530 U.S. 428, 120 S. Ct. 2326 (2000).

enforcement agencies and courts to follow.'"[11] Those guidelines mandate the administration of [the] warnings which have now "come to be known colloquially as '*Miranda* rights.'"[12] The *Miranda* warnings, held the Dickerson Court, are constitutional in dimension; the warnings have "become embedded in routine police practice to the point where the warnings have become part of our national culture."[13]

An accused certainly may, of course, waive his or her *Miranda* rights, provided the waiver is made *voluntarily, knowingly, and intelligently*.[14] A law enforcement official's failure to abide by *Miranda's* procedural safeguards—the administration of the warnings and receipt of an appropriate waiver—renders any and all statements obtained from an accused in any ensuing custodial interrogation inadmissible at trial, at least in the prosecution's case-in-chief.[15]

§7.3. The Formula

From the foregoing discussion, it is clear that prior to any custodial interrogation, law enforcement officers are required to administer the *Miranda* warnings to the person about to be questioned. The formula should be as easy as 1 + 1 = 2; that is, *"custody"* + *"interrogation"* = *the requirement* that *Miranda* warnings be given.[16] For law enforcement, the desired, ultimate result is the acquisition of a valid confession, fully admissible at trial. For that to occur, officers are at all times required to scrupulously honor each of the rights contained within the *Miranda* warnings.[17]

---

[11] *Id.*, 120 S. Ct. at 2331.
[12] *Id.*
[13] *Id.*, 120 S. Ct. at 2335-36.
[14] *Miranda v. Arizona*, 384 U.S. 436, 444-45, 86 S. Ct. 1602, 1612 (1966).
[15] *See Michigan v. Tucker*, 417 U.S. 433, 444, 94 S. Ct. 2357, 2364 (1974) (recognizing that *Miranda's* "procedural safeguards were not themselves rights protected by the Constitution but were instead measures to insure that the right against compulsory self-incrimination was protected").
[16] *See generally* Larry E. Holtz, *Interviews, Confessions and Miranda: Cases and Materials* (Training Manual for classes held in 2017 and 2018).
[17] *Id.*

§7.4. Volunteered Statements

"Not all admissions or confessions obtained in the absence of *Miranda* warnings are inadmissible. The formula set forth in the preceding section — *custody* + *interrogation* = the requirement that *Miranda* warnings be given — teaches that law enforcement officials may, without the administration of *Miranda* warnings, question a criminal suspect who is not in custody. Moreover, officers may utilize any admission or confession volunteered by an in-custody criminal suspect when no interrogation (express or implied) has taken place.[18] In this respect, the Court in *Miranda* emphasized that "[a]ny statement given freely and voluntarily without any compelling influences is, of course, admissible in evidence."[19] Law enforcement officials are by no means required to stop people from speaking when they step forward to confess to a crime. Volunteered statements of any kind are not barred by the Fifth Amendment and their admissibility has not been affected by the Court's ruling in *Miranda*.[20]

§7.5. Custody in General

In *Miranda*, the Supreme Court defined "custodial interrogation" as "questioning initiated by law enforcement officers after a person has been taken into custody or otherwise deprived of his freedom of action in any significant way."[21] Deciding whether a person is in custody for purposes of *Miranda* is an objective determination, based on all the surrounding circumstances. It is determined on the basis of "how a reasonable person in the suspect's situation would perceive his circumstances."[22]

---

[18] *Id.*
[19] *Miranda v. Arizona*, 384 U.S. 436, 478, 86 S. Ct. 1602, 1630 (1966).
[20] *Rhode Island v. Innis*, 446 U.S. 291, 300-01, 100 S. Ct. 1682 (1980); *see also United States v. Beckwith*, 22 F. Supp.2d 1270 (D.Utah 1998); *State v. Kell*, 61 P.3d 1019 (Utah 2002).
[21] *Miranda v. Arizona*, 384 U.S. 436, 444, 86 S. Ct. 1602, 1612 (1966); *see also Stansbury v. California*, 511 U.S. 318 (1994).
[22] *Yarborough v. Alvarado*, 541 U.S. 652, 662, 124 S. Ct. 2140, 2148 (2004); *see also Stansbury v. California*, 511 U.S. 318, 323, 114 S. Ct. 1526, 1529 (1994) (The "initial determination of custody depends on the objective circumstances of the interrogation, not on the subjective views harbored by either the interrogating officers or the person being questioned.").

"Custody," for purposes of *Miranda*, has also been described as "a term of art that specifies circumstances that are thought generally to present a serious danger of coercion. In determining whether a person is in custody in this sense, the initial step is to ascertain whether, in light of the objective circumstances of the interrogation, a reasonable person would have felt he or she was not at liberty to terminate the interrogation and leave."[23]

To determine whether an interrogation is custodial, courts will consider such factors as:[24]

(1) The time, place and physical surroundings of the questioning;

(2) The nature and degree of the pressure applied to detain the individual;

(3) The duration and mode of the questioning and/or detention;

(4) The conduct and language used by the police in dealing with the individual;

(5) The number of law enforcement officers present;

(6) Whether there were members of the person's family or friends present;

(7) The age, intelligence and mental condition of the subject; and

(8) Whether the person was advised that he was not under arrest and was free to leave.

For juveniles, the United States Supreme Court in *J.D.B. v. North Carolina*[25] held that the *Miranda* custody analysis should also include a consideration of the juvenile suspect's age. "[S]o long as the child's age was known to the officer at the time of police questioning, or would have been objectively apparent to a reasonable officer, its inclusion in the custody analysis is consistent with the objective

---

[23] *Howes v. Fields*, 565 U.S. 499, 132 S. Ct. 1181, 1189 (2012) (citations and internal quotes omitted).

[24] *See generally J.D.B. v. North Carolina*, 564 U.S. 261, 131 S.Ct. 2394 (2011); *United States v. Booth*, 669 F.2d 1231 (9th Cir. 1981); *State v. Timmendequas*, 161 N.J. 515, 614, 737 A.2d 55 (1999); *State v. Galloway*, 133 N.J. 631, 654, 628 A.2d 735 (1993); *see also Schneckloth v. Bustamonte*, 412 U.S. 218, 226, 93 S.Ct. 2041, 2047-48 (1973).

[25] *J.D.B. v. North Carolina*, 564 U.S. 261, 131 S.Ct. 2394 (2011).

Admissions and Confessions 173

nature of that test. This is not to say that a child's age will be a determinative, or even a significant, factor in every case."[26] "Just as police officers are competent to account for other objective circumstances that are a matter of degree such as the length of questioning or the number of officers present, so too are they competent to evaluate the effect of relative age. * * * In short, officers and judges need no imaginative powers, knowledge of developmental psychology, training in cognitive science, or expertise in social and cultural anthropology to account for a child's age. They simply need the common sense to know that a 7-year-old is not a 13-year-old and neither is an adult."[27]

At the stationhouse. In *Oregon v. Mathiason*,[28] the Supreme Court held that *Miranda* warnings are not required when law enforcement officers question a suspect who is neither under arrest nor "in custody" when such questioning takes place within the confines of the police station house. According to the Court, "police officers are not required to administer *Miranda* warnings to everyone whom they question. Nor is the requirement of warnings to be imposed simply because the questioning takes place in the station house, or because the questioned person is one whom the police suspect. *Miranda* warnings are required only where there has been such a restriction on a person's freedom as to render him 'in custody.'"[29]

§7.6. Interrogation in General

The Court in *Miranda* suggested that "interrogation" referred only to actual "questioning initiated by law enforcement officers."[30] There are times, however, when a creative and inventive officer may overpower the will of the individual questioned *without asking any questions whatsoever*. It is this type of "psychological ploy" that necessarily undermines the privilege against compulsory self-incrimination, and, such ploys may thereby be treated as the

---

[26] *J.D.B.*, 131 S. Ct. at 2406 (citing, for example, teenagers nearing age 18).
[27] *Id.* at 2407.
[28] 429 U.S. 492, 97 S. Ct. 711 (1977).
[29] *Id.*, 97 S. Ct. a 714; see also *California v. Beheler*, 463 U.S. 1121, 103 S. Ct. 3517 (1983).
[30] *Miranda v. Arizona*, 384 U.S. 436, 444, 86 S. Ct. 1602, 1612 (1966).

"functional equivalent" of interrogation.[31] Thus, to determine whether an "interrogation" has taken place, courts will examine whether the police used any words or actions that they *knew or should have known* were "reasonably likely to elicit an incriminating response from the suspect."[32] After the initiation of formal charges, the critical question will be whether officers *deliberately elicited* incriminating information from a defendant in the absence of counsel after a formal charge against the defendant had been filed.[33]

In *Rhode Island v. Innis*,[34] the Supreme Court addressed the police use of a psychological ploy to prompt an admission from a suspect after his arrest but before any formal charges had been filed (a time period known as the "Fifth Amendment" setting). Since there was no direct questioning of the suspect, the Court examined whether the suspect's incriminating response, in this Fifth Amendment setting, was or was not the product of "any words or actions on the part of the police (other than those normally attendant to arrest and custody) that the *police should know are (or should have known were) reasonably likely to elicit an incriminating response from the suspect.*"[35] "Incriminating response" refers to "any response—whether inculpatory or exculpatory—that the prosecution may seek to introduce at trial." The *reasonably-likely-to-elicit standard* thus "focuses primarily upon the perceptions of the suspect, rather than the intent of the police." A practice that the police should know is reasonably likely to evoke an incriminating response from a suspect thus amounts to interrogation.

In *Innis*, the police were investigating the murder of a taxicab driver. He had died from what appeared to be a shotgun blast to the back of his head. The day after the driver's body was found, the police received a call from another taxicab driver reporting that he had just been robbed by a "man wielding a sawed-off shotgun." After the driver identified defendant from a photo lineup, the police began searching for him.

---

[31] *See generally* Larry E. Holtz, *Interviews, Confessions and Miranda: Cases and Materials* (Training Manual for classes held in 2017 and 2018).
[32] *Rhode Island v. Innis*, 446 U.S. 291, 301, 100 S. Ct. 1682, 1689-90 (1980).
[33] *Massiah v. United States*, 377 U.S. 201, 206, 84 S. Ct. 1199, 1203 (1964).
[34] *Rhode Island v. Innis*, 446 U.S. 291, 100 S. Ct. 1682 (1980).
[35] *Id.*, 446 U.S. 291, 100 S. Ct. 1682, 1689-90 (emphasis added).

Within a few hours, defendant was spotted, arrested, and advised of his *Miranda* rights. Defendant stated that he understood his rights and wanted to speak to an attorney. The officers then placed defendant in a "caged wagon," a four-door police car with a wire screen mesh between the front and rear seats, and drove him to headquarters. During the ride to the police station, the following conversation took place among the officers:

> I frequent this area while on patrol and there's a lot of handicapped children running around in this area, and God forbid one of them might find a weapon with shells and they might hurt themselves . . . it would be too bad if the little girl would pick up the gun, maybe kill herself.[36]

Defendant then interrupted the conversation and requested that the officers turn the patrol car around so he could show them where the gun was located. Defendant stated that he understood his rights, but he "wanted to get the gun out of the way because of the kids in the area in the school." Defendant then directed the police to a nearby field and pointed out the hidden shotgun.[37]

According to the Court, because defendant's incriminating response was not the product of words or actions of the police that they *should have known were reasonably likely to elicit an incriminating response*, their actions did not constitute "interrogation" within the meaning of Miranda.[38]

Once the individual has been formally charged with an offense, the courts apply a stricter approach to define "interrogation," asking whether the police "deliberately elicited" incriminating statements. In *Brewer v. Williams*,[39] the famous "Christian Burial" case, the Supreme Court held that defendant Williams was "interrogated" in violation of his Sixth Amendment right to counsel.

---

[36] *Id.*, 446 U.S. at 294-95, 110 S. Ct. at 1686-87.
[37] *Id.* at 295, 110 S.Ct. at 1687.
[38] *Id.* 446 U.S. at 303, 100 S. Ct. at 1691.
[39] *Brewer v. Williams*, 430 U.S. 387, 97 S. Ct. 1232 (1977).

The facts unfolded on the afternoon of December 24, when 10-year-old Pamela Powers went with her family to the YMCA in Des Moines, Iowa, to watch a wrestling tournament in which her brother was participating. When she failed to return from a trip to the bathroom, an unsuccessful search for her began.

Robert Williams, who had recently escaped from a mental hospital, was a resident of the YMCA. Soon after the girl's disappearance, Williams was seen leaving the YMCA carrying some clothing and a large bundle wrapped in a blanket. He placed the large bundle in his car and drove off. His abandoned car was found the following day in Davenport, Iowa, roughly 160 miles east of Des Moines. A warrant was then issued in Des Moines for his arrest on a charge of abduction.

On the morning of December 26, acting on the advice of an attorney, Williams turned himself in to the Davenport police, where he was booked on the charge specified in the arrest warrant. After advising Williams of his *Miranda* rights, the Davenport police telephoned representatives of the Des Moines Police Department and advised them that Williams had surrendered. At the time, Williams' attorney was still at Des Moines police headquarters. The attorney spoke with Williams on the telephone and advised him that Des Moines officers would be driving to Davenport to pick him up and that the officers would not interrogate him. Prior to the trip, Williams was arraigned before a judge in Davenport on the outstanding arrest warrant.

Detective Leaming and his fellow officer arrived in Davenport at about noon to pick up Williams and return him to Des Moines. The two detectives, along with Williams, then set out on the 160-mile drive. Leaming knew that Williams was a former mental patient and knew also that he was deeply religious. Not long after leaving Davenport and reaching the interstate highway, Detective Leaming addressed Williams as "Reverend," and said:

> I want to give you something to think about while we're traveling down the road .... Number one, I want you to observe the weather conditions, it's raining, it's sleeting, it's freezing, driving is very treacherous, visibility is poor, it's

going to be dark early this evening. They are predicting several inches of snow for tonight, and I feel that you yourself are the only person that knows where this little girl's body is, that you yourself have only been there once, and if you get a snow on top of it, you yourself may be unable to find it. And, since we will be going right past the area on the way into Des Moines, I feel that we could stop and locate the body, that the parents of this little girl should be entitled to a Christian burial for the little girl who was snatched away from them on Christmas Eve and murdered. And I feel we should stop and locate it on the way in, rather than waiting until morning and trying to come back out after a snow storm and possibly not being able to find it at all.[40]

As they continued toward Des Moines, just as they approached Mitchellville, Williams said that he would show the officers where the body was. He then directed the police to the body of Pamela Powers.

Holding that Williams was "interrogated," the Court said: The police detective "deliberately and designedly set out to elicit information from Williams just as surely as — and perhaps more effectively than — if he had formally interrogated him." The detective's "Christian burial speech" was "tantamount to interrogation."[41] Because the detective did not obtain from Williams a waiver of his right to counsel prior to that "interrogation," neither Williams' incriminating statements themselves nor any testimony describing his having led the police to the victim's body can constitutionally be admitted into evidence.[42]

---

[40] *Id.* at 392-93, 97 S. Ct. at 1236.
[41] *Id.* at 400, 97 S.Ct. at 1240.
[42] *Id. See also Fellers v. United States,* 540 U.S. 519, 524, 124 S. Ct. 1019, 1022 (2004) (reaffirming application of the "deliberate-elicitation standard" for Sixth Amendment cases). In a subsequent court proceeding, the evidence related to the body of 10-year-old Pamela Powers was ultimately determined to be admissible. As Detective Leaming drove Williams to Des Moines, a large-scale search party consisting of two hundred volunteers had been combing the area. The detectives called off the search when they believed Williams would lead them to the little girl's body. The child's body was found in a ditch beside a gravel road in Polk County about two miles south of Interstate 80. The location was essentially within the area to be searched. In fact, the body was found approximately two and one-half miles from where the search had stopped. The Court held that, under the "inevitable discovery rule," the evidenced would have been ultimately or inevitably discovered by lawful means. *See Nix v. Williams,* 467 U.S. 431, 104 S.Ct. 2501, 2509 (1984).

§7.7. *Miranda* and On-the-Scene Questioning

General on-the-scene questioning as to facts surrounding a crime or other general questioning of citizens in the fact-finding process is not affected by the *Miranda* decision.[43]

§7.8. *Miranda's* "Public Safety" Exception

In *New York v. Quarles*,[44] the Supreme Court created a *"public safety exception"* to the requirement that *Miranda* warnings be administered before a suspect's answers may be admitted into evidence. The Court determined that the need for answers to questions in situations which pose a significant threat to the public safety justify a law enforcement officer's delay in advising an arrestee of his *Miranda* rights.

In *Quarles*, officers were stopped while on patrol by a woman who advised the officers that she was just raped. The woman provided a particularized description of the suspect and further stated that he ran into a supermarket located nearby and was carrying a gun. The officers located the suspect in the supermarket and proceeded to stop and frisk him. The frisk revealed a concealed shoulder holster, which was empty. At that point, the officers placed the suspect under arrest, handcuffed him, and then asked him one question: "Where is the gun?" The arrestee motioned to the gun's location and the officers immediately recovered a loaded .38 caliber revolver from an empty carton. At this point the officers read the arrestee his *Miranda* rights.

The Court held that the circumstances in this case presented overriding considerations of public safety to justify the officers' failure to administer *Miranda* warnings before they asked a question

---

[43] *See Miranda v. Arizona*, 384 U.S. 436, 477, 86 S.Ct. 1602, 1629 (1966); *see also State v. Gosser*, 50 N.J. 438, 446 (1967) (In addition to recognizing that uncoerced, freely-volunteered statements are admissible at trial even in the absence of *Miranda*, courts also recognize an exception to the *Miranda* exclusionary rule, which permits the introduction of a suspect's responses to an officer's "on-the-scene questioning as to the facts surrounding a crime.").

[44] *New York v. Quarles*, 467 U.S. 649, 104 S. Ct. 2626 (1984).

devoted to locating the abandoned gun. "Public safety must be paramount to adherence to the literal language of the prophylactic rules enunciated in *Miranda*." Here, the police were presented with the immediate necessity of ascertaining the location of a gun which they had every reason to believe the suspect had just removed from his holster and discarded in the supermarket. So long as the gun was concealed somewhere in the supermarket, with its whereabouts unknown, it posed many significant dangers to the public safety. Administration of *Miranda* in such circumstances might deter a suspect from responding and have a result of creating a significant danger to the public—that of a concealed loaded gun in a public area.

Under the public safety exception, an officer may also ask about the presence of dangerous objects on a suspect's person before frisking the suspect without violating *Miranda*.

§7.9. Asserting the Right to Silence or the Right to Counsel

(a) *The right to remain silent.* Once a suspect invokes his or her right to remain silent, all questioning must stop. The Court in *Miranda* did not, however, decide whether, and under what circumstances, law enforcement authorities may resume questioning the suspect. In *Michigan v. Mosley*,[45] the Court revisited this issue and noted that a strict, literal reading of the phrase "all questioning must cease" would lead to "absurd and unintended results."[46] The Mosley Court concluded that *Miranda* did not impose an absolute ban on the resumption of questioning following an invocation of the right to remain silent by a person in custody. The Court held that "the admissibility of statements obtained after the person in custody has decided to remain silent depends under *Miranda* on whether his right to cut off questioning was scrupulously honored."[47] Mosley's expression of his desire to remain silent was deemed "scrupulously honored" based on the facts that: (1) Mosley had been advised of his *Miranda* rights before both interrogations; (2) the officer conducting

---

[45] *Michigan v. Mosley*, 423 U.S. 96, 96 S. Ct. 321 (1975).
[46] *Mosley*, at 102, 96 S. Ct. at 325.
[47] *Id.* at 102-03, 96 S. Ct. at 326.

the first interrogation immediately ceased all questioning when Mosley expressed his desire to remain silent; (3) the second interrogation occurred after a significant time lapse; (4) the second interrogation was conducted in another location; (5) by another officer; and (6) it related to a different offense.

One person cannot assert another person's right to remain silent. Exercising one's right to remain silent is, in effect, asserting one's Fifth Amendment privilege to be free from self-incrimination. As noted by the United States Supreme Court in *Bellis v. United States*,[48] "the Fifth Amendment privilege is purely a personal one."[49] Thus, it has been held that one person may not assert another person's right to be free from self-incrimination.[50] This limitation on the Fifth Amendment, as affording an entirely personal right, has been understood among the courts to support the conclusion that the Fifth Amendment "cannot be asserted vicariously."[51] Note that a different result may occur when a caregiver of a person with special needs indicates that the person cannot respond.

(b) *The right to counsel.* When an in-custody suspect requests counsel, all questioning must stop. This was made clear by the Supreme Court in *Edwards v. Arizona.*[52] *Edwards* held that once a suspect invokes the right to counsel, "a valid waiver of that right cannot be established by showing only that he responded to further *police initiated* custodial interrogation even if he has been advised of his rights."[53]

The assertion of a suspect's right to an attorney while being questioned in police custody is "an invocation of his Fifth Amendment rights, requiring that all interrogation must cease."[54] If the accused indicates in any manner that he may desire a lawyer, the

---

[48] 417 U.S. 85, 94 S. Ct. 2179 (1974).
[49] *Bellis* at 90, 94 S.Ct. at 2184.
[50] *See, e.g., State v. Baum,* 199 N.J. 407, 419-420, 972 A.2d 1127, 1133-34 (2009).
[51] *See United States v. Fortna,* 796 F.2d 724, 732 (5th Cir. 1986); *United States v. Ward,* 989 F.2d 1015, 1020 (9th Cir.1992) (concluding that defendant "had no standing to assert the ... Fifth Amendment rights of others"); *State v. Ducharme,* 601 A.2d 937, 941 (R.I. 1991) ("One may not complain about compulsion that may be applied to another.").
[52] *Edwards v. Arizona,* 451 U.S. 477, 101 S. Ct. 1880 (1981).
[53] *Edwards* at 484-85, 101 S. Ct. at 1884-85.
[54] *Edwards* at 485, 101 S. Ct. at 1885.

police may not ask him any further questions or reinitiate questioning "until counsel has been made available to him, *unless the accused himself initiates further communication, exchanges or conversations with the police.*"[55] In these circumstances, courts will question first whether the accused invoked his right to counsel. If so, the inquiry next addresses whether the accused or the police initiated further communications or exchanges about the investigation.

If it is determined that the police initiated further questioning after a previous assertion of the right to counsel, any statements made by the accused will be inadmissible at trial unless, at the time of the second or subsequent questioning, the accused had been given an opportunity "to confer with [an] attorney and to have him present during" the second or subsequent questioning session.[56] If, however, it is determined that the accused himself initiated further communication, exchanges or conversations about the investigation, the inquiry would then be whether, after providing the accused with a fresh set of *Miranda* warnings, the police received "a valid waiver of the right to counsel and the right to silence[,]" that is, whether the accused voluntarily, knowingly and intelligently waived his rights based on "the totality of the circumstances, including the necessary fact that the accused, not the police, reopened the dialogue with the authorities."[57]

In *Smith v. Illinois*,[58] the Court pointed out that, on occasion, an accused's asserted request for counsel may be ambiguous or equivocal. But in this case, no one has pointed to anything Smith previously had said that might have cast doubt on the meaning of his statement, "I'd like to do that," upon learning that he had the right to his counsel's presence. Nor is there anything in that statement itself, which would suggest anything inherently ambiguous or equivocal. "Where nothing about the request for counsel or the circumstances leading up to the request would render it ambiguous, all questioning must cease."

---

[55] *Id.* (emphasis added).
[56] *Id. See also Minnick v. Mississippi*, 498 U.S. 146, 111 S. Ct. 486, 491 (1990) ("when counsel is requested, interrogation must cease, and officials may not reinitiate interrogation without counsel present, whether or not the accused has consulted with his attorney").
[57] *Edwards* at 486 n.9, 101 S. Ct. at 1885 n.9.
[58] *Smith v. Illinois*, 469 U.S. 91, 105 S. Ct. 490 (1984).

However, in *Davis v. United States*,[59] the Court held that defendant's "remark to the NIS agents— 'Maybe I should talk to a lawyer'— was not a request for counsel." Consequently, the NIS agents "were not required to stop questioning [defendant], though it was entirely proper for them to clarify whether [defendant] in fact wanted a lawyer."[60] The Court wrote, "after a knowing and voluntary waiver of the *Miranda* rights, law enforcement officers may continue questioning until and unless the suspect *clearly requests* an attorney."

It has been held, however, that if, before waiving his or her *Miranda* rights, the suspect gives a response to questioning that is ambiguous but may be construed as invoking either the right to remain silent or the right to counsel, the officers conducting the interrogation may only ask questions designed to clarify the suspect's intent and determine whether, in fact, the suspect wishes to invoke his or her *Miranda* rights.

The Shatzer 14-day rule. In *Maryland v. Shatzer*,[61] the Supreme Court held that once the suspect has been released from *Miranda* custody for *14 days*, the police may reapproach the suspect and ask whether he is now willing to answer questions. According to the Court, a 14-day period "provides plenty of time for the suspect to get reacclimated to his normal life, to consult with friends and counsel, and to shake off any residual coercive effects of his prior custody."[62]

Recall that in *Edwards v. Arizona*, the Court created a *presumption* that once a suspect invokes the *Miranda* right to counsel, any waiver of that right in response to a subsequent police attempt at custodial interrogation is *involuntary*. The *Edwards* presumption is designed to prevent the police from badgering a suspect into waiving his or her previously asserted *Miranda* rights.

In the typical case, the suspect is arrested and is held in uninterrupted pretrial custody while the crime is being actively

---

[59] *Davis v. United States*, 512 U.S. 452, 114 S. Ct. 2350 (1994).
[60] *Id.*, 512 U.S. 452, 114 S. Ct. at 2357.
[61] *Maryland v. Shatzer*, 559 U.S. 98, 130 S. Ct. 1213 (2010).
[62] *Id.* at 110, 130 S. Ct. 1213, 1223 (2010).

investigated. While *Edwards* did not address whether this rule survives a break in custody, lower courts have uniformly held that a break in custody ends the *Edwards* presumption. In *Shatzer*, the Court held: "[L]aw enforcement officers need to know, with certainty and beforehand, when renewed interrogation is lawful. And while it is certainly unusual for this Court to set forth precise time limits governing police action, it is not unheard-of."[63] Accordingly, 14 days is an appropriate period of time to avoid the consequence of the Edwards presumption. "That provides plenty of time for the suspect to get reacclimated to his normal life, to consult with friends and counsel, and to shake off any residual coercive effects of his prior custody."[64]

§7.10. Waiver of Rights

To be valid, a criminal defendant's waiver of his or her rights must be made voluntarily, knowingly, and intelligently, and the government bears the burden of proof. Under the federal Constitution, the prosecution must prove waiver by a "preponderance of the evidence."[65] When a court assesses the voluntariness of a waiver of rights, it considers the characteristics of the suspect and the totality of the circumstances surrounding the interrogation. Relevant factors will include, but not be limited to:

- the suspect's age, education, intelligence and mental condition.
- the suspect's background, experience and any previous encounters with law enforcement.
- how and by what method the suspect was advised of his constitutional rights.
- the length of the detention.
- the period of time between administration of *Miranda* warnings and any statement given.

---

[63] *Id.* at 110, 130 S.Ct. at 1222-23.
[64] *Id.*
[65] *Colorado v. Connelly*, 479 U.S. 157, 107 S. Ct. 515, 523 (1986).

- the nature of the questioning and whether it was repeated or prolonged.
- whether physical or mental punishment, coerciveness, or mental exhaustion was involved.
- whether the suspect was deprived of food, sleep or medical attention.
- whether the suspect was injured, intoxicated or drugged, or in ill health.
- Whether law enforcement officials made an express promise of leniency or sentence.[66]

(a) *Voluntariness—a two-step analysis.* As a general proposition, the admissibility of a confession depends on whether it was voluntarily made. "The ultimate issue is whether the confession was the product of an essentially free and unconstrained choice by its maker. 'If it is, if he has willed to confess, it may be used against him. If it is not, if his will has been overborne and his capacity for self-determination critically impaired, the use of his confession offends due process.'"[67] Unlike the use of physical coercion, however, use of psychologically oriented methods during questioning are not inherently coercive. The critical inquiry in such cases is whether the person's decision to confess results from a free and self-directed choice rather than from an overbearing of the suspect's will.[68] A court's inquiry into waiver has two distinct dimensions: (1) the relinquishment of the right must have been voluntary in the sense that it was the product of free and deliberate choice rather than

---

[66] *See Colorado v. Connelly,* 479 U.S. 157, 107 S. Ct. 515, 522 (1986); *see also Schneckloth v. Bustamonte,* 412 U.S. 218, 226, 93 S. Ct. 2041, 2047-48 (1973); *State v. Hreha,* 217 N.J. 368, 383, 89 A.3d 1223, 1231-32 (2014).

[67] *Arizona v. Fulminante,* 499 U.S. 279, 111 S. Ct. 1246, 1261 (1991) (quoting *Culombe v. Connecticut,* 367 U.S. 568, 602, 81 S. Ct. 1860, 1879 (1961)); *see also Blackburn v. Alabama,* 361 U.S. 199, 206, 80 S. Ct. 274, 279 (1960) ("coercion can be mental as well as physical, and* * *the blood of the accused is not the only hallmark of an unconstitutional inquisition").

[68] *See Arizona v. Fulminante,* 499 U.S. 279, 111 S. Ct. 1246, 1252-53 (1991) (confession held involuntary where defendant, an alleged child murderer in danger of physical violence from other inmates, was motivated to confess when a fellow inmate (a government agent) promised to protect him in exchange for the confession); *Payne v. Arkansas,* 356 U.S. 560, 561, 78 S. Ct. 844, 846 (1958) (confession held to be coerced because the interrogating officer had promised that if the accused confessed, the officer would protect him from an angry mob outside the jailhouse door).

Admissions and Confessions

intimidation, coercion or deception; and (2) the waiver must have been made with a full awareness of both the nature of the right being abandoned and the consequences of the decision to abandon it.

(b) *A free and unconstrained choice; inducements to confess.* Police are not permitted to employ unreasonable or improper inducements that impair a suspect's decision whether to give a statement or seek legal counsel. The rule applies to those situations where the police prompt an admission or confession by suggesting a benefit if the suspect forgoes his or her rights. This reasoning was first announced in *Bram v. United States*,[69] where the United States Supreme Court declared: "[A] confession, in order to be admissible, must be free and voluntary: that is, [it] must not be extracted by any sort of threats of violence, nor obtained by any direct or implied promises, . . . nor by exertion of any improper influence[.]"[70] Involuntariness may also be shown by an express promise of leniency, such as the police telling the defendant that, in return for his cooperation, his punishment would be less severe. Clearly, "threats of physical violence" will "render involuntary a confession obtained thereafter."[71]

A knowing and intelligent choice. The question of whether a waiver of rights was the product of force, threat, duress, improper influence, or any other type of coercive police activity is only half the equation. The second step in the inquiry questions whether the waiver was given "knowingly and intelligently." Among other things, this requires that the administration of the *Miranda* warnings be more than a mere perfunctory exercise. This second aspect requires that the defendant comprehend the plain meaning of his basic *Miranda* rights. Here, the prosecution will be asked to show that any such waiver was not only knowing and voluntary, but that the suspect understood the right that he or she was waiving.

(c) *Lying to a suspect.* Lying to a suspect will not, by itself, render a confession involuntary. The lie may not, however, be the sole motivating factor for the suspect's decision to confess. For example,

---

[69] *Bram v. United States*, 168 U.S. 532, 542-43, 18 S. Ct. 183, 187 (1897).
[70] *Id.*
[71] *See, e.g., Lynum v. Illinois*, 372 U.S. 528, 537, 83 S. Ct. 917 (1963) (defendant's confession involuntary when police told her that her state financial aid would be cut off and her six children taken from her unless she "cooperated" with them).

in *Frazier v. Cupp*,[72] the United States Supreme Court held that the defendant's confession was admissible notwithstanding the fact that the police falsely told him that another person had confessed. The Court noted that the defendant was a mature person of normal intelligence and that the questioning session lasted only slightly over an hour.[73] In *Frazier*, the police falsely told a defendant that his codefendant had already confessed. The court concluded that "the fact that the police misrepresented the statements [the codefendant] had made is, while relevant, insufficient in our view to make this otherwise voluntary confession inadmissible."[74]

Similarly, in *Bobby v. Dixon*,[75] the Court held that the defendant's confession, which was obtained by urging defendant to "cut a deal" before his accomplice did so, was lawfully obtained. According to the Court, the police tactic used was common and constitutional.

Telling defendant that the information is vitally needed for the victim's medical treatment. In *State v. Galloway*,[76] Galloway admitted shaking his girlfriend's three-month-old child very hard several times, thereby injuring the child and causing his eventual death. At the hospital's emergency room, the interrogating officer told defendant that the baby was seriously injured, and asked Galloway to describe exactly what he had done to the baby so the doctors could treat the child accordingly. The Court described the officer's conduct as "a deliberate act of deception to secure a confession." Nonetheless, the Court ruled that (1) the officer's actions did not rise to an improper level of psychological pressure warranting suppression of defendant's confession; and (2) the defendant's confession "was the result of a knowing, voluntary, and intelligent waiver" of his rights.

---

[72] 394 U.S. 731, 89 S. Ct. 1420 (1969).
[73] *Frazier* at 739, 89 S. Ct. at 1425.
[74] *Id.*
[75] 565 U.S. 23, 28, 132 S.Ct. 26, 29 (2011); *see also Oregon v. Elstad*, 470 U.S. 298, 317, 105 S. Ct. 1285, 1297 (1985) ("[T]he Court has refused to find that a defendant who confesses, after being falsely told that his codefendant has turned State's evidence, does so involuntarily.").
[76] 133 N.J. 631, 628 A.2d 735 (1993).

The Court said:

> The police had no reason to believe that defendant would be particularly vulnerable to interrogation. At the time of the arrest, defendant was twenty-seven years old. He had a tenth-grade education, but had received a G.E.D. Psychological testing shows that defendant's IQ is "dull normal." Defendant had served in the Army for three years[, and he] had some minimal experience with the police, from a prior arrest and conviction for writing bad checks. Moreover, at the police station, defendant was not deprived of food or drink. Defendant saw his father, albeit in the presence of the police. Although defendant may not have slept that night, he did not appear tired. Defendant appeared to be under stress and was crying. However, the fact that defendant was distressed and emotional is not by itself sufficient to render his confession involuntary. [And he] was repeatedly told pursuant to *Miranda* that whatever he said would be used against him.[77]

Cases holding that misrepresentations by law enforcement were improper generally also contained police conduct that had overborne the will of the defendant. Such cases have typically required a showing of very substantial psychological pressure on the defendant. For example, in *Darwin v. Connecticut*,[78] the Court held that defendant's will was overborne when he was kept from speaking to an attorney or other persons for thirty to forty-eight hours. In *Clewis v. Texas*,[79] the Court determined that defendant's will was overborne when officers subjected defendant (with a fifth-grade education) to thirty-eight hours of intermittent interrogation and did not notify him of his right to an attorney. Here, the Court also noted the possibility of the defendant being deprived of food, sleep and human contact. Similarly, in *Gallegos v. Colorado*,[80] the Court held that the defendant's will was overborne after officers detained the fourteen-year-old for five days during which time he saw no lawyer, parent, or other friendly adult.

---

[77] *Id.* at 656-57, 628 A.2d at 748.
[78] 391 U.S. 346, 88 S.Ct. 1488 (1968).
[79] 386 U.S. 707, 87 S.Ct. 1338 (1967).
[80] 370 U.S. 49, 82 S.Ct. 1209 (1962).

(d) *Juveniles and intellectually impaired individuals.* A knowing and intelligent waiver of *Miranda* also means that the suspect had the ability to understand the very words used in the warnings. It need not mean the ability to understand far-reaching legal and strategic effects of waiving one's rights, or to appreciate how widely or deeply an interrogation may probe, or to withstand the influence of stress or fancy; but to waive rights intelligently and knowingly, one must at least understand basically what those rights encompass and minimally what their waiver will entail.[81]

Miranda warnings with simplified explanations. Law enforcement officials will find the following "Youth Rights Form" to be very helpful in dealing with intellectually impaired defendants, as well as juveniles.[82]

YOUTH RIGHTS FORM

Youth/Person in custody: _____. Age: _____. DOB: _____.
Place: _____ Date: _____.
Day of week: _____. Time child/person taken into custody: _____.
Time this form was read: _____. Official: _____.
Parent (Guardian or Custodian) present: _____.
        [If other than parent, indicate relationship.]

Parent (Guardian or Custodian) not present.___ Unable to contact after ___ attempts.
                            [Check]   [Number]
[See last page for times and places of contact attempts.]; or _____ contact made,
                                                             [Check]
unwilling to attend.

[The following must be read and explained by the officer, and the youth and parent, guardian, or custodian) shall read it before signing.]

---

[81] *See* Larry E. Holtz, *Miranda in a Juvenile Setting: A Child's Right to Silence*, 78 J. Crim. L. & Criminology 534, 536-37, 546-56 (1987) (citing evidence that most youths lack proper comprehension of rights under police interrogation; providing a simplified version of Miranda warnings—a "Youth Rights Form"). *Compare Reno v. Flores*, 507 U.S. 292, 113 S. Ct. 1439, 1451 (1993) ("juveniles are capable"—at least 16- and 17-year-olds— "of 'knowingly and intelligently' waiving their right against self-incrimination") (citing *Fare v. Michael C.*, 442 U.S. 707, 724-27, 99 S. Ct. 2560, 2571-73 (1979), and *United States v. Saucedo-Velasquez*, 843 F.2d 832, 835 (5th Cir. 1988) (applying Fare to an alien juvenile)).

[82] Larry E. Holtz, *Miranda in a Juvenile Setting: A Child's Right to Silence*, 78 J. Crim. L. & Criminology 534, 536-37, 546-56 (1987)

Admissions and Confessions

Before I am allowed to ask you any questions, you must understand that you have certain important rights, or protections, that have been given to you by our laws in these situations. These rights will make sure that you will be treated fairly. You will not be punished for deciding to use these rights. I will read these rights to you, and explain each of them to you if you don't understand them, or think you may not understand them. You may ask questions as we go along so that you can completely understand what your rights are.

Do you understand me so far? Yes _____. No _____.
Parent (Guardian or Custodian) Yes _____. No _____.

1. You have the right to remain silent or the right to talk to us about this matter. This means that you do not have to write or say anything; not with me or anyone else, not now or later on. You will not be punished for deciding not to talk to us.

Do you understand this right? Yes _____. No _____.
Parent (Guardian or Custodian) Yes _____. No _____.

2. If you give up your right to remain silent, anything you say can and may be used against you in court. This means that if you decide to talk to me or answer questions, I can go to court and tell the judge what you said. This also means that if you say or write anything, what you say or write can be used in a court to prove that you may have broken the law.

Do you understand this? Yes _____. No _____.
Parent (Guardian or Custodian) Yes _____. No _____.

2a. You have the right to have your parent, guardian, or custodian present here with you before we talk to you or ask you any questions. This means that before we ask you anything about this matter, you can, and should, call your parents (guardian or custodian) so they can be here with you to help you.

Do you understand this right? Yes _____. No _____.

3. You have a right to talk to an attorney, a lawyer, before any questioning. You have the right to have the lawyer here with you while you are being questioned. The lawyer will help you. If you decide that you want a lawyer, we will not question you or talk to you at all until you speak to the lawyer and have him here with you.

Do you understand this right? Yes _____. No _____.
Parent (Guardian or Custodian) Yes _____. No _____.

4. You have the right to stop talking to us at any time. You also have the right to ask for a lawyer to be here with you at any time. This means that if you decide, at any time during questioning, that you do not want to talk anymore, you may tell us to stop and we will not ask you any more questions. Also, if you decide you would like to talk to a lawyer at any time during questioning, you will not

be asked any more questions until a lawyer is here with you and you have talked with him.

Do you understand this right?   Yes _____. No _____.
Parent (Guardian or Custodian)   Yes _____. No _____.

5. If you want to talk to a lawyer and you and your family do not have the money to pay for one, you can still have a lawyer for free before any questioning about this matter begins.

Do you understand this right?   Yes _____. No _____.
Parent (Guardian or Custodian)   Yes _____. No _____.

6. [For serious crimes only] There is a possibility that you may not be brought to juvenile court, but, instead, will be treated as an adult in an adult criminal court. If that happens, the procedures—the way your case will be handled—will be different. However, you will still keep and have all the rights I have explained to you. You must also understand that anything you may say to me by talking with me or answering my questions could be used to decide whether you are treated as a juvenile or as an adult. If you are to be treated as an adult, we, or the court, will explain the adult procedures and results which could include jail or prison if you are found guilty.

Do you understand this?   Yes _____. No _____.
Parent (Guardian or Custodian)   Yes _____. No _____.

7. You must always understand that if you decide to exercise or use any or all of your rights, you will not be hurt or punished in any way at all. These are your rights and my rights and our laws give them to you and me in the same way.

Do you have any questions so far? Yes _____. No _____.
Parent (Guardian or Custodian)   Yes _____. No _____.

If yes (nature of question): _____
_____
_____
_____

[The Official should make sure the following portion is read by the youth.]

8. I can read and understand English. Yes _____. No _____.
   I go to school.   No _____. Yes _____;
                                      Present Grade _____.

Admissions and Confessions 191

ATTORNEY REQUEST

After listening to my rights and reading my rights, I fully understand what my rights are. At this time I would like to have a lawyer.

Signature of Youth: _____. Date _____. Time _____.
Signature of Parent (Guardian or Custodian): _____
Signature of Official: _____

GUARDIAN OR CUSTODIAN

EXPLAIN NATURE OF RELATIONSHIP AND SOURCE OF THE GUARDIAN'S OR CUSTODIAN'S AUTHORITY TO "GUIDE" OR "COUNSEL" THE YOUTH IN THIS CASE, AND WHETHER THE GUARDIAN OR CUSTODIAN HAS "LEGAL CUSTODY" OF THE YOUTH.

_____
_____

WAIVER

I have been read and I have read my rights as listed above. I fully understand what my rights are. I am willing to give up my right to remain silent. I am willing to answer questions. I give up my right to have a lawyer present. I do not wish to speak to a lawyer before I answer any questions. No promises or threats or special offers have been made to me to make me give up my rights. I understand that I may change my mind at any time and say that I want to use my rights. I also understand that if I change my mind, it will not affect what I have already said or done.

Signature of Youth: _____.
Signature of Parent (Guardian or Custodian): _____.
Witness [Type or Print]: _____.
Signature of Witness: _____. Telephone: _____.
Official's Name [Type or Print]: _____. Date: _____.
Signature of Official: _____. Time: _____.
_____

DOCUMENTATION OF OFFICIAL ATTEMPTS TO CONTACT PARENT (GUARDIAN OR CUSTODIAN) OF YOUTH

Date: _____. Time: _____.
Method: _____
Response: _____

Date: _____. Time: _____.
Method: _____
Response: _____

Date: _____. Time: _____.
Method: _____
Response: _____

Date: _____. Time: _____.
Method: _____
Response: _____

(e) *Intoxicated suspects.* Suspects who are in pain, intoxicated or on drugs may not be able to give a knowing, intelligent and voluntary waiver. In such cases, the prosecution has the burden of showing by a preponderance of the evidence that the waiver was voluntary, knowing and intelligent.[83]

(f) *Persons with dementia.* In *Miller v. State*,[84] Miller claimed that his confession should have been suppressed on voluntariness grounds, asserting that his mental impairments, specifically his early signs of dementia, should have been obvious. In rejecting his claim, the Supreme Court of Florida concluded that Miller "fully understood his *Miranda* rights."[85] Said the court:

> Miller has prior experience with the law and exposure to the *Miranda* warnings. "The crucial test is whether the words in the context used, considering the age, background and intelligence of the individual being interrogated, impart a clear, understandable warning of all of his rights." ... Miller's background and knowledge of law enforcement demonstrate that he understood the warnings with regard to his rights. In fact, he expressly stated to law enforcement that he normally would not talk to police and would first to talk to an attorney, but was going to "do something that he had never done before." Thus, Miller expressed a willingness to talk that was premised on his prior understanding that he had a right to an attorney, which is a right he normally utilized. When the warnings given to Miller are considered in context with his age, background, and intelligence, they imparted a clear, understandable warning of all of his rights."

---

[83] *Colorado v. Connelly*, 479 U.S. 157 (1986).
[84] 161 So.3d 354 (Fla. 2015).
[85] *Id.* at 372.

This conclusion is supported by the mental health experts' evaluations of Miller, none of whom concluded that the results of the MRI or their neurological evaluations indicated that his neurological impairments prohibited him from making a knowing, voluntary, and intelligent waiver of his *Miranda* rights. In fact, Dr. Mings testified during the evidentiary hearing that the defense specifically retained him to determine whether Miller was competent to waive his *Miranda* rights. Dr. Mings conducted an "Assessing, Understanding, and Appreciation of *Miranda* Rights" questionnaire and determined that Miller "made very few, if any, errors on that. He understood all of the questions, [and] answered them appropriately."[86]

In an unpublished decision out of California, the court in *People v. Schoenhofen*,[87] addressed the defendant's contention that the trial court erred by concluding that he knowingly and intelligently waived his *Miranda* rights during his police interview. Defendant, James Schoenhofen, pointed out that, at the time of the police questioning, he was 67 years old, suffered from dementia and other medical and psychological problems, had not slept much the night before, had not received food since breakfast the day of the interview, and had not received any of his prescribed medications.

After conducting an independent review of the one-hour recorded interview, the California Court of Appeal held that "the totality of circumstances establishes that Schoenhofen's waiver of his *Miranda* rights was knowing, intelligent, and voluntary. Schoenhofen stated that he was 67 or 68, adding that his birthday was several weeks away. Although Schoenhofen did not know his cellular telephone number, he explained that he acquired the telephone recently and his wife possessed it. He also stated that he recently moved to a rural desert area and did not know his street address." In addition, "Schoenhofen stated that he had two community college degrees and discussed his employment history and medical and psychological problems. Following the *Miranda* advisements, he stated that he might 'not answer all the questions.' Schoenhofen later

---

[86] *Id.* at 372-73 (quoting *Coyote v. United States*, 380 F.2d 305, 308 (10th Cir. 1967)).
[87] 2014 Cal. App. Unpub. LEXIS 3712.

stated that he would not submit to a polygraph test. He also expressed anger regarding execution of the search warrant [at his] home. Schoenhofen responded to [the officer's] questions, admitted certain improper acts with M. and K.B., but insisted that he did not commit other improper acts. He asked Escalante to define child molestation and expressed surprise that possession of child pornography is illegal." Further, the court's review of the recorded interview revealed that the officer instructed Schoenhofen to provide an audible response to the *Miranda* advisements, when she asked if he could "say yes." Accordingly, in view of the totality of circumstances, the court held that Schoenhofen's waiver was knowing, voluntary, and intelligent.

Thus, simply because a person may be suffering from mild dementia or possesses a low IQ does not necessarily mean that the person cannot knowingly and intelligently waive his or her *Miranda* rights. To this end, courts have found several instances where defendants, despite certain mental impairments, have waived their rights knowingly and intelligently.[88]

In *Garner v. Mitchell*,[89] the court reviewed the assessments of the Garner's doctors, all of whom indicated that Garner suffered from diminished mental capacity, a troubled upbringing, and a poor education at the time that he confessed to his crimes. According to the court, however, these assessments did not demonstrate that

---

[88] *See, e.g., United States v. Turner*, 157 F.3d 552, 555 (8th Cir. 1998) (holding that a defendant's borderline IQ did not prevent a knowing and intelligent waiver); *Rice v. Cooper*, 148 F.3d 747, 749, 750-51 (7th Cir. 1998) (holding that a mildly retarded defendant gave a valid waiver because police had no reason to suspect that he did not understand the warnings); *Correll v. Thompson*, 63 F.3d 1279, 1288 (4th Cir. 1995) (finding that a defendant's waiver of his *Miranda* rights was knowing and intelligent despite the fact that the defendant possessed an IQ of only 68 because he was 24 years old and had previously had numerous experiences with law enforcement and *Miranda* warnings). See also *People v. Ratcliff*, 2015 Cal. App. Unpub. LEXIS 10900 ("[R]egardless of whether defendant may have suffered from some degree of dementia, she appeared to have no significant difficulty in understanding the detective's explanation of the *Miranda* rights or any other aspect of the questioning. To the contrary, her statements were coherent and responsive and gave every objective indication that she well understood what was being asked of her, and freely chose to make a statement.").

[89] 557 F.3d 257 (6th Cir. 2009).

Admissions and Confessions 195

Garner "was incapable of knowingly and intelligently waiving his *Miranda* rights."[90] In this regard, the court instructed:

> It is well-established, in this circuit and others, that mental capacity is one of many factors to be considered in the totality of the circumstances analysis regarding whether a *Miranda* waiver was knowing and intelligent. Thus, diminished mental capacity alone does not prevent a defendant from validly waiving his or her *Miranda* rights.[91]

Thus, mental capacity is simply one factor that must be viewed alongside other factors, including evidence of the defendant's conduct during, and leading up to, the interrogation. Case law in other circuits is instructive in this regard.

(g) *Persons with intellectual disabilities.* In *Smith v. Mullin*,[92] the Tenth Circuit held that the defendant's *Miranda* waiver was knowing and intelligent despite the facts that (1) the defendant suffered from borderline mental retardation, and (2) a clinical psychologist had concluded, based on the defendant's Grisso[93] test scores, that the

---

[90] *Id.* at 264.

[91] *Id.* at 264-65 (citing *Clark v. Mitchell*, 425 F.3d 270, 283-84 (6th Cir. 2005) (holding that in the context of the voluntariness of a confession, the Sixth Circuit concluded that "borderline retardation" or "low average intellect" was not dispositive on the question of voluntariness); *United States v. Rojas-Tapia*, 446 F.3d 1, 7-9 (1st Cir. 2006); *Smith v. Mullin*, 379 F.3d 919, 933-34 (10th Cir. 2004); *Young v. Walls*, 311 F.3d 846, 849 (7th Cir. 2002); *United States v. Turner*, 157 F.3d 552, 555-56 (8th Cir. 1998); *Rice v. Cooper*, 148 F.3d 747, 750 (7th Cir. 1998); *Henderson v. DeTella*, 97 F.3d 942, 948-49 (7th Cir. 1996); *Correll v. Thompson*, 63 F.3d 1279, 1288 (4th Cir. 1995); *Starr v. Lockhart*, 23 F.3d 1280, 1294 (8th Cir. 1994); *Derrick v. Peterson*, 924 F.2d 813, 824 (9th Cir. 1991); *Toste v. Lopes*, 861 F.2d 782, 783 (2d Cir. 1988); *Dunkins v. Thigpen*, 854 F.2d 394, 399-400 (11th Cir. 1988).

[92] 379 F.3d 919 (10th Cir. 2004).

[93] Dr. Thomas Grisso developed a testing instruments—*Instruments for Assessing Understanding and Appreciation of Miranda Rights*—which were designed to measure an examinee's basic understanding of the *Miranda* warnings, as well as the examinee's appreciation of the significance of the warnings in police, legal and court proceedings. Although the Grisso instruments have been used by a number of experts in the field, the instrument has several limitations. First, the instrument provides only an estimate of the examinee's understanding and appreciation of his or her rights at the time of the evaluation. Questions about the validity of a *Miranda* waiver typically are not raised at the time the waiver is offered, and a great deal of time may pass between the waiver and the evaluation. Thus, the examinee's understanding and appreciation of the *Miranda* rights may have changed in the interim as a result of discussions with the attorney,

defendant could not have validly waived his rights.[94] The Tenth Circuit found it significant that the clinical psychologist also testified that the defendant "would understand the role of police officers and the concept of a criminal charge," and that the Grisso test was administered years after the interrogation.[95] The court also relied on a videotape showing the defendant's conduct during the interrogation and noted that the defendant had had previous experience with the criminal justice system.[96]

In *United States v. Turner*,[97] the Eighth Circuit held that the defendant's *Miranda* waiver was knowing and intelligent even though the defendant's IQ was low-average to borderline, and he was possibly intoxicated by PCP at the time of interrogation and exhibited "bizarre" behavior and possible signs of mental illness after the interrogation.[98] The court determined that because the defendant was cooperative during the interrogation, gave accurate information, and, when stopped by police, "acted in a manner more consistent with a person attempting to avoid being caught than a person who did not know what he was doing," the waiver was effective.[99]

In some cases, courts have concluded that a defendant's limited intellectual capacity contributed to the determination that a waiver was not effective. Frequently, however, those cases also feature some observable indication to police that the defendant was incapable of

---

maturation, or experience.

Furthermore, although the instrument provides information about capacities related to the knowing and intelligent requirements of a valid *Miranda* waiver, they do not measure the validity of the waiver. Rather, the evaluator can use data from the instruments to inform the court about an examinee's capacities to understand and appreciate his or her rights. The court may then use this information, in conjunction with other factors considered in the totality of circumstances test, to determine the ultimate question of waiver validity. *See also* Bruce Frumkin and Martin Sellbom, *Miranda Rights Comprehension Instruments (MRCI); A Critical Review*, (2013), presenting a revision of Grisso's original series of tests. According to the authors, the MRCI represents an improvement in many respects, including (but not limited to) a thorough discussion of admissibility issues in the test manual, simplification of language, the addition of a fifth warning, and updated normative data.

[94] *Id.* at 932-34.
[95] *Id.* at 933.
[96] *Id.* at 934.
[97] 157 F.3d 552 (8th Cir. 1998).
[98] *Id.* at 555-56.
[99] *Id.* at 555.

Admissions and Confessions 197

understanding the *Miranda* warnings. For example, in *United States v. Garibay*,[100] the defendant suffered from a low IQ, but also primarily spoke Spanish and thus did not possess the English skills to understand the *Miranda* warnings without the assistance of a Spanish-speaking officer. Additionally, an officer that questioned the defendant was forced to rephrase questions when the defendant "did not appear to understand."[101] In *Cooper v. Griffin*,[102] the Fifth Circuit held that neither defendant knowingly and intelligently waived his *Miranda* rights where both defendants were young boys, aged fifteen and sixteen, who were severely mentally retarded.

In the *Garner* case, Garner's conduct, speech, and appearance at the time of interrogation indicated that his waiver was knowing and intelligent, notwithstanding his diminished mental capacity. Like the defendants in *Mullin* and *Turner*, Garner was carefully read his *Miranda* rights and stated clearly to officers that he understood those rights. Garner agreed to execute a written waiver form, was cooperative during the interrogation, and clearly explained the incident[.] Garner also engaged in conduct prior to being arrested that was "more consistent with a person attempting to avoid being caught than a person who did not know what he was doing."[103] Garner invented a story about having a fight with his girlfriend to explain to the taxicab driver why he was removing the items from [the victim's] apartment, and Garner admitted to police that his purpose in lighting the couch on fire was to ensure that he left no fingerprints behind. Finally, "at no time did Garner exhibit any outwardly observable indications that he did not understand the warnings or the circumstances surrounding his interrogation. Garner was not a minor, did not have trouble understanding English, and, although his IQ level indicates that he was functioning in the borderline range of intelligence, he was not so mentally retarded that officers had reason to believe that he could not understand his rights."[104]

---

[100] 143 F.3d 534, 537-38 (9th Cir. 1998).
[101] *Id.* at 539.
[102] 455 F.2d 1142, 1144-46 (5th Cir. 1972).
[103] *See, e.g., Turner*, 157 F.3d at 555.
[104] *Garner* at 266. In the following cases, waivers were found to be valid. *United States v. Macklin*, 900 F.2d 948 (6th Cir. 1990) (defendant had IQ of 59; co-defendant's IQ was 70); *Moore v. Dugger*, 856 F.2d 129 (11th Cir. 1988) (defendant had IQ of 62 and

When a law enforcement officer prepares to question a person who may have dementia, or who may be demonstrating some form of mental impairment or intellectual disability, the officer should consider the following:

- Approaching the individual in a calm, nonthreatening manner. Introduce yourself and be respectful;

- Give the person some space, don't touch the individual. You do not want to appear threatening;

- If you are in a noisy area consider moving to a quieter one with fewer distractions;

- Electronically recording the interview, if feasible;

- Securing the attendance of an interested adult or advocate to assist the individual;

- Carefully reading the *Miranda* rights and using language that is easy to understand;

- Assessing whether the person's conduct, speech, and appearance at the time of questioning indicate that the person has the ability to knowingly and intelligently waive their *Miranda* rights, notwithstanding a possible diminished mental capacity.

---

functioned on the level of eleven-year-old child); *Reddix v. Thigpen,* 805 F.2d 506 (5th Cir. 1986) (intellectually impaired defendant); *De La Rosa v. Texas,* 743 F.2d 299 (5th Cir. 1984) (borderline intellectually impaired defendant); *Harris v. Riddle,* 551 F.2d 936 (4th Cir. 1977) (IQ of 67; sixth grade intelligence); *United States v. Young,* 529 F.2d 193 (4th Cir. 1975) (below average IQ; limited education and reading ability); *Hill v. State,* 303 Ark. 462, 798 S.W.2d 65 (Ark. 1990) (IQ between 56 and 70; third grade functioning); *State v. Brooks,* 648 So. 2d 366 (La. 1995) (borderline intellectual disability, but functional); *State v. Cook,* 175 W. Va. 185, 332 S.E.2d 147 (W. Va. 1985) (moderate intellectual impairment).

Conversely, in the following cases, statements were suppressed. *Henry v. Dees,* 658 F.2d 406 (5th Cir. 1981) (IQ between 65 and 69; sixth-grade level of education); *Cooper v. Griffin,* 455 F.2d 1142 (5th Cir. 1972) (defendants with IQs between 61 and 67; low functioning); *State v. Flower,* 224 N.J. Super. 208, 539 A.2d 1284 (N.J. Super. Ct. Law Div. 1987) (IQ less than 70; mental age equivalency of seven to twelve-year-old child).

- Assessing whether the person's conduct on being taken into custody demonstrated proper behavior that was more consistent with a person attempting to avoid being caught than a person who did not know what he was doing.

- Assessing whether the person's conduct shows signs of mental impairment; whether the person makes any inappropriate comments; or acts in a way that would lead you to believe that he or she is confused, delusional, or unable to understand you.

When you begin to question the suspect, do so in a calm voice, don't talk loudly; don't yell. Tell them that you are just going to talk to them. Be kind, introduce yourself. Tell them you are going to sit with them and ask some questions. The questions that follow are designed to assist you in determining whether the person is aware of their surroundings, i.e., oriented to time and place, and whether the person has special needs. The questions are basic and could be answered by the average person. They determine language comprehension, cognitive processing, the ability to carry out simple commands, basic reading, math and writing skills.

This process can determine the person's basic abilities. Recognize that if a person with special needs is experiencing extreme fear and stress they may not be able to answer the questions due to confusion and anxiety. How many times have you heard, "I am so upset, I can't think!" This happens to average people and happens more frequently to people with disabilities. Allow some time to pass and try again. If they do not respond, they may just be noncompliant and disrespectful, or there may be other reasons. They may not speak English; they may be deaf; they may be so stressed that they can't respond. You may have to repeat the question. You may need an interpreter for the deaf or a language interpreter before you can proceed.

- Assessing whether the person can answer a few simple questions will help you determine the person's ability to cognitively process simple commands. Take careful notes so you can include this information in your report.

- You can ask all or some of the following sample questions:
  - ~ What is your name?
  - ~ What day is it?
  - ~ What time of day is it?
  - ~ Please read this card with your rights aloud.
    (Purpose: This will determine if the person can read.)

- Ask the person to:
  - ~ Tell me two things you do in the morning.
    (Purpose: Anything they say is relevant, don't correct them. Typical responses are: go to the bathroom, brush teeth, shower, or eat breakfast. Any atypical response should be noted.)

- Hand the person a sheet of blank paper and a pen or pencil. Ask the person to:
  - ~ Sign your first name on this piece of paper.
    (Purpose: This will determine if the person can write in cursive. If the person prints their name, or writes in large, immature letters, this indicates the person's educational level. If, however, the person has a physical disability, for example, cerebral palsy, they may be unable to physically manage this.)
  - ~ Draw a triangle, a square and a circle.
    (Purpose: This will determine if the person comprehends the shapes. Observe their grasp of the pen, is it typical? This will determine if the person is able to remember three items, which tests their short-term memory.)
  - ~ Count backwards from the number 20.
    (Purpose: This indicates simple number knowledge.)
  - ~ How many is in a dozen?
    Wait for the answer, then ask, "If you have a dozen eggs and six eggs break, how many are left?" (Note that if the person originally says 13, ask why. They may be talking about a "baker's dozen," which is, in fact 13.) (Purpose: Mathematical reasoning and problem solving.)
  - ~ Can you count by odd numbers?
    (Purpose: This indicates a basic understanding of math concepts.)

Admissions and Confessions 201

> ~ Who is the President of the United States?
> (Purpose: This indicates an understanding of current events.)
> ~ What state are we in?
> ~ What are the seasons of the year?
> Wait for the answer, then ask, what season is it now?
> (Purpose: Indicates an awareness of time and place.

The individual may ask, "Did I get that right?" They may need positive reinforcement, so give them reassurance. Say, "You are doing a good job." If this happens, you just received essential information about the person's capacity. It tells you that they may be guessing and not know the answers to your questions. Whatever their response, do not correct them. The information you are obtaining needs to go into your report. After the question and answer period is over, thank them for helping you and being cooperative. Many of these individuals need continuous positive reassurance; they may have faced past learning experiences that were negative.

The Affirmative Dilemma. There may be an instance when a person is questioned and he or she consistently responds with "Yes!" Recognize at this point that the person may not know the answer and may just be trying to please you or simply cooperate. In their mind, they believe they may be doing the right thing.

Here is an extreme example:

Q. *Do you understand the rights I just read to you?*
   A. Yes.
Q. *Do you want to waive your rights?*
   A. Yes.
Q. *Do you need a pen?*
   A. Yes.
Q. *Can you write your name?*
   A. Yes.
Q. *Did you kill the victim?*
   A. Yes.
Q. *What is the victim's name?*
   A. Yes.

Q. *Is the victim Jimmy Hoffa?*
A. Yes.
Q. *Is Jimmy Hoffa related to Big Bird?*
A. Yes.

At this point, it is obvious there is a problem. What is happening is "the *Affirmative Dilemma,*" whereby the person is answering "yes" to everything. Stop your questioning. At this point, you can assume the person is not competent and does not understand their *Miranda* rights.

For example, in *State v. Flower,*[105] twenty-six-year-old defendant Flower was charged with first degree aggravated sexual assault upon a 3½-year-old child. Upon his arrest, he was given the *Miranda* warnings by a prosecutor's investigator. Defendant admitted that the confession he gave was not the product of physical or mental force or coercion, but instead, indicated that he was "afraid of going to jail" so he answered every question yes. The record demonstrated that defendant had the limited intelligence of a six- or seven-year-old child and an IQ of less than 70. The evidence introduced at the hearing revealed that defendant "had to be spoken to in very basic terms and any instructions given to him had to be repeated time and again and also repeated by him before one could be certain that he understood. His limited vocabulary was of a second- or third-grade level, and he was described as not having the ability to grasp and understand concepts or abstractions."[106] At court, it became "readily and quickly apparent to the judge that defendant did not know his right hand from his left, could not see from his right eye, and could neither read nor write. A foster guardian with whom defendant resided for the past seven years testified that defendant would 'say yes to anything.'"[107]

In light of these circumstances, the court held that the prosecution failed to prove that defendant "knowingly and intelligently" waived his *Miranda* rights because he simply could not understand

---

[105] 224 *N.J.Super.* 208, 539 A.2d 1284 (Law Div. 1987), *aff'd mem.*, 224 *N.J.Super.* 90 (App.Div. 1988).
[106] *Id.* at 211.
[107] *Id.* at 211-12.

Admissions and Confessions

them. "One cannot knowingly and intelligently waive a right that he cannot understand or appreciate."[108]

This is a prime example of a jurisdiction that treats an accused with diminished mental capacity (whether because of age or a mental defect) differently than it does adults who are presumed to be responsible. The former holds a protected status in our society. "Therefore, when ascertaining whether a person with diminished mental capacity acted knowingly and intelligently, the court must satisfy itself that the administering of constitutional rights was more than a mere perfunctory procedure."[109]

Bear in mind that there are some disabled individuals who are very intelligent, but are ill-equipped socially and have very low emotional intelligence. They may do quite well on the questions and appear bright and articulate. Yet they are awkward in situations and could easily be persuaded by others to participate in inappropriate or illegal activities to gain social acceptance.

The questions outlined in this section may be used at any time to help a law enforcement officer determine very rudimentary and basic functional capabilities of an individual. While they seem to be very simple, remember that the measurement of intellectual capacity and emotional intelligence is not an exact science. The methods are meant as a simple, quick guide to assist the officer in dealing with an individual with special needs. It is not a measurement device but a simple quick reference to help determine if an advocate is needed for an individual with special needs.

Recognize that the person may have difficulty with verbal communication. That does not mean that they do not understand. Individuals with intellectual disabilities may understand what you are saying—this is *receptive* language—but may not be able to verbally respond—this is *expressive* language.

Also recognize that the courts have held that a person's mental capacity is only one factor in determining whether someone's waiver

---

[108] *Id.* at 216, 539 A.2d at 1287.
[109] *Id.* at 216, 539 A.2d at 1287; *see also State v. Cleary*, 161 Vt. 403, 413, 641 A.2d 102, 108 (1994).

of *Miranda* rights was voluntary, knowing and intelligent. Just as in the law of consent, a person is not precluded from waiving his or her rights "simply because he or she suffers from a mental disease."[110]

Be sure to document the nuances of the interview. Having this record (written, audio or video) will provide you and others with a general baseline of the individual's ability. Determining whether an individual has a disability is a difficult task. Added to that difficulty is the fact that law enforcement officers out in the field many times need to make split-second decisions in tense, rapidly evolving situations. Keep in mind that an individual with a disability may act out or behave differently than others at the scene. Be alert to those differences and document them as required.

§7.11. Outside Influences

Often in the interrogation process, factors outside or extrinsic to the actual questioning session may work to undermine the integrity of the process or the voluntariness of the defendant's responses. How an officer deals with such outside influences will, in many cases, determine the admissibility of any statements the defendant may make. For example, in *Colorado v. Connelly*,[111] the Supreme Court held that a suspect's confession will not be deemed to be "involuntary" on Due Process grounds when it results from the suspect's internal compulsion caused by a mental illness rather than from police overreaching. Connelly confessed to killing an individual because, as he stated to the police officer, "his conscience was bothering him," and "voices told him to confess." The Court held this to be a valid confession, for "coercive police activity,"

---

[110] *See United States v. Richards*, 741 F.3d 843, 846-47 (7th Cir. 2014); *see also State v. Blackstock*, 19 S.W.3d 200, 208 (Tenn. 2000) (" '[N]o single factor, such as IQ, is necessarily determinative in deciding whether a person was capable of knowingly and intelligently waiving, and does so waive, the constitutional rights embraced in the *Miranda* rubric.'") (quoting *Fairchild v. Lockhart*, 744 F. Supp. 1429, 1453 (E.D. Ark. 1989)). "Among the circumstances courts have considered are the defendant's age, background, level of functioning, reading and writing skills, prior experience with the criminal justice system, demeanor, responsiveness to questioning, possible malingering, and the manner, detail, and language in which the *Miranda* rights are explained. As a result, courts tend to reach results that are somewhat fact-specific." *Blackstock* at 208.

[111] 479 U.S. 157, 107 S. Ct. 515 (1986).

which was not present in the case, "is a necessary predicate to the finding that a confession is not 'voluntary' within the meaning of the Due Process Clause of the Fourteenth Amendment."[112]

The Deity Dilemma. The *Deity Dilemma* refers to those situations where persons confess as a result of some religious necessity or due to a message received from some omnipotent being. For example, in January 2018, a man confessed to the 1993 stabbing murder of a 19-year-old. Brian Hawkins said that he was "sick of running" and that "God and Christ" and his own conscience had pushed him to confess. After announcing his involvement in the crime to a local news agency, he walked next door into the sheriff's department and confessed. [113]

---

[112] *Id.* at 167, 107 S. Ct. at 522.
[113] https://www.uproxx.com/news/brian-keith-hawkins-confess-cold-case-murder

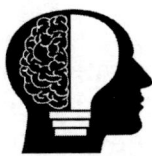

KEY POINTS

- Properly secured admissions and confessions are integral in the law enforcement scheme and are extremely persuasive at trial.

- The introduction of an admission or a confession at trial is like no other evidence. The defendant's own confession is probably the most probative and damaging evidence that can be admitted against him.

- Prior to custodial interrogation, the person must be informed of their *Miranda* rights:

  - You have the right to remain silent.
  - Anything you say can and will be used against you in a court of law.
  - You have the right to consult with an attorney and have an attorney present during questioning.
  - If you cannot afford an attorney, one can be provided to you before questioning at no cost.
  - You may ask for an attorney at any time during questioning, and questioning will stop if at any time you ask for an attorney.

- Volunteered statements of any kind are not barred by the Fifth Amendment and their admissibility has not been affected by the Court's ruling in *Miranda*.

KEY POINTS (Continued)

- After the advice of rights, if the individual indicates in any manner and at any stage of the process that he wishes to consult with an attorney before speaking there can be no questioning. Likewise, if the individual is alone and indicates in any manner that he does not wish to be interrogated, the police may not question him.

- Consideration must be given to the juvenile suspect's age when objectively apparent to a reasonable officer.

- Officers and judges need no imaginative powers, knowledge of developmental psychology, training in cognitive science, or expertise in social and cultural anthropology to account for a child's age. They simply need common sense.

- To be valid, a criminal defendant's waiver of his or her rights must be made voluntarily, knowingly, and intelligently, and the government bears the burden of proof.

- A knowing and intelligent waiver of *Miranda* also means that the suspect had the ability to understand the very words used in the warnings. It need not mean the ability to understand far-reaching legal and strategic effects of waiving one's rights, or to appreciate how widely or deeply an interrogation may probe, or to withstand the influence of stress or fancy; but to waive rights intelligently and knowingly.

- *Miranda warnings with simplified explanations.* Law enforcement officials will find the "Youth Rights Form," (located in this chapter) very helpful in dealing with intellectually impaired defendants and juveniles.

KEY POINTS (Continued)

- In some cases, courts have concluded that a defendant's limited intellectual capacity contributed to the determination that a waiver was not effective. Frequently, however, those cases also feature some observable indication to police that the defendant was incapable.

- Simply because a person may have mild dementia or possesses a low IQ does not necessarily mean that the person cannot knowingly and intelligently waive his or her *Miranda* rights.

- When an officer prepares to question a person who may have dementia, or who may be demonstrating some form of mental impairment or intellectual disability, the officer should consider the following:

    ~ Approaching the individual in a calm, nonthreatening manner. Introduce yourself and be respectful.

    ~ Not getting too close; give the person some space, don't touch the individual.

    ~ If you are in a noisy area consider moving to a quieter one with fewer distractions.

    ~ Electronically recording the interview, if feasible.

    ~ Securing the attendance of an interested adult or advocate to assist the individual.

    ~ Carefully reading the *Miranda* rights and using language that is easy to understand.

KEY POINTS (Continued)

~ Assessing whether the person's conduct, speech and appearance at the time of questioning indicate that the person has the ability to knowingly and intelligently waive their *Miranda* rights, notwithstanding a possible diminished mental capacity.

~ Assessing whether the person's conduct on being taken into custody demonstrated proper behavior that was more consistent with a person attempting to avoid being caught than a person who did not know what he was doing.

~ Assessing whether the person's conduct shows signs of mental impairment; whether the person makes any inappropriate comments; or acts in a way that would lead you to believe that he or she is confused, delusional, or unable to understand you.

Chapter Eight
OBTAINING CONSENT TO SEARCH

§8.1. Introduction

When a person consents to a search of his property, he gives up his or her constitutional right to be free from unreasonable searches and seizures. A "consent to search" procedure is treated by the courts as a recognized exception to the written warrant requirement. As such, consensual searches continue to provide law enforcement officials with access to those areas in which an officer, desirous of searching, does not have probable cause to conduct a constitutional search or to secure a warrant. When a search is conducted pursuant to a valid consent, it may be conducted without a warrant and without probable cause.[1]

To be valid, a person's consent must be provided "voluntarily," "knowingly," and "intelligently."[2] First and foremost, the consent must be voluntary; included in this requirement, the consent must be unequivocal and specific. Mere acquiescence cannot substitute for free consent. When consent is voluntary, it is freely and intelligently given, uncontaminated by any duress or coercion, actual or implied.

In all cases, "the question whether a consent to a search was in fact 'voluntary' or was the product of duress or coercion, express or implied, is a question of fact to be determined from the totality of the circumstances."[4] Moreover, under the Fourth Amendment and in most states, the prosecution has the burden of proof to show by a preponderance of the evidence that the consent to search was freely and voluntarily given.[5] Some states, however, are more demanding

---

[1] *United States v. Matlock*, 415 U.S. 164, 165, 94 S. Ct. 988, 990 (1974); *Schneckloth v. Bustamonte*, 412 U.S. 218, 222, 93 S. Ct. 2041, 2045 (1973).
[2] *Bumper v. North Carolina*, 391 U.S. 543, 548, 88 S. Ct. 1788 (1968).
[3] *Judd v. United States*, 89 U.S. App. D.C. 64, 66, 190 F.2d 649, 651 (D.C. Cir. 1951).
[4] *Schneckloth v. Bustamonte*, 412 U.S. 218, 227, 93 S. Ct. 2041, 2047-48 (1973).
[5] *Schneckloth v. Bustamonte*, 412 U.S. 218, 227, 93 S. Ct. 2041, 2047-48 (1973).

and require a higher standard. For example, in New Jersey, the courts require the State to prove a voluntary, knowing and intelligent consent by clear and positive evidence.[6]

As aptly observed by the United States Supreme Court:

> "Consent searches are part of the standard investigatory techniques of law enforcement agencies" and are "a constitutionally permissible and wholly legitimate aspect of effective police activity." It would be unreasonable—indeed, absurd—to require police officers to obtain a warrant when the sole owner or occupant of a house or apartment voluntarily consents to a search. The owner of a home has a right to allow others to enter and examine the premises, and there is no reason why the owner should not be permitted to extend this same privilege to police officers if that is the owner's choice. Where the owner believes that he or she is under suspicion, the owner may want the police to search the premises so that their suspicions are dispelled. This may be particularly important where the owner has a strong interest in the apprehension of the perpetrator of a crime and believes that the suspicions of the police are deflecting the course of their investigation. An owner may want the police to search even where they lack probable cause, and if a warrant were always required, this could not be done. And even where the police could establish probable cause, requiring a warrant despite the owner's consent would needlessly inconvenience everyone involved—not only the officers and the magistrate but also the occupant of the premises, who would generally either be compelled or would feel a need to stay until the search was completed.[7]

Law enforcement officials are not permitted to employ unreasonable or improper inducements that impair a suspect's decision whether to provide consent to search. The rule applies to those

---

[6] *See, e.g., State v. King*, 44 N.J. 346, 352, 209 A.2d 110, 113 (1965) (Consent must be "voluntary"—"freely and intelligently given," and "[t]he burden of proof is on the State to establish by clear and positive testimony that the consent was so given.").

[7] *Fernandez v. California*, 571 U.S. ___, 134 S. Ct. 1126, 1132 (2014) (quoting *Schneckloth v. Bustamonte*, 412 U.S. 218, 228, 231-32, 93 S. Ct. 2041, 2045 (1973)).

situations where the police obtain consent to search by suggesting a benefit if the suspect forgoes his or her rights. In addition, involuntariness may be shown by an express promise of leniency, such as an officer telling the subject that, in return for his cooperation, his punishment would be less severe.

§8.2. The Right to Refuse Consent

Under the United States Constitution (and numerous state constitutions as well), there is no requirement that officers tell an individual he or she has a right to refuse permission to search. "The law today is that knowledge of the right to refuse is but one factor in the totality of the circumstances to be examined in construing the reasonableness of a search."[8] This interpretation of the Fourth Amendment is not always followed, however. For example, in New Jersey, it has been held that knowledge of the right to refuse is an essential element of voluntary consent under the state constitution.[9]

Similarly, some states have held that an officer may not engage in a "knock and talk" without advising the homeowner of the "right to refuse."[10] A "knock and talk" procedure is a law enforcement tactic by which the police, who possess some information that they believe warrants further investigation, but that is insufficient to constitute probable cause for a search warrant, approach the person suspected of engaging in illegal activity at the person's residence (even knock on the front door), identify themselves as police officers,

---

[8] *Schneckloth v. Bustamonte,* 412 U.S. 218, 227, 93 S. Ct. 2041, 2047-48 (1973).

[9] *See, e.g., State v. Johnson,* 68 N.J. 349, 353-54, 346 A.2d 66, 68 (1975) ("We conclude that under Art. I, par. 7 of our State Constitution the validity of a consent to a search, even in a non-custodial situation, must be measured in terms of waiver; i.e., where the State seeks to justify a search on the basis of consent it has the burden of showing that the consent was voluntary, an essential element of which is knowledge of the right to refuse consent."); *see also State v. Carty,* 170 N.J. 632, 639, 790 A.2d 903. 907 (2002).

[10] *See, e.g., State v. Ferrier,* 136 Wn.2d 103, 118-119, 960 P.2d 927, 934 (1998) ("When police officers conduct a knock and talk for the purpose of obtaining consent to search a home, and thereby avoid the necessity of obtaining a warrant, they must, prior to entering the home, inform the person from whom consent is sought that he or she may lawfully refuse to consent to the search and that [he or she] can revoke, at any time, the consent that [he or she] gives, and can limit the scope of the consent to certain areas of the home. The failure to provide these warnings, prior to entering the home, vitiates any consent given thereafter.").

and request consent to search for the suspected illegality or illicit items. Courts have upheld that "knock and talk" procedure, for the officer may approach a home and knock, precisely because that is "no more than any private citizen might do."[11]

§8.3. Determining Whether the Consent Was Voluntary or Coerced

There are several factors that a court will examine to determine whether a consent was voluntarily given or coerced. Factors which may suggest that consent was coerced include:

(1) the presence of abusive, overbearing, or dictatorial police procedures;

(2) police use of psychological ploys, or subtle psychological pressure or language, or a tone of voice that indicated compliance with the request might be compelled;

(3) statements or acts on the part of the police that convey to the consenting party that he was not free to refuse the search or to walk away from the officer;

(4) that consent was obtained despite the consenting party's denial of guilt;

(5) that consent was obtained only after the consenting party had refused initial requests for consent to search;

(6) that consent was given after the police blocked or otherwise impaired the consenting party's progress, or in some other way physically restrained the individual, for example, by the use of handcuffs, by surrounding the individual with uni-

---

[11] *Florida v. Jardines*, 569 U.S. 1, 6, 8, 133 S. Ct. 1409, 1415 (2013); *see also Carroll v. Carman*, 574 U.S. ___, 135 S.Ct. 348, 351 (2014) (open to the suggestion that an unsuccessful attempt at a "knock and talk" visit at the front door does not automatically prohibit officers from trying the back door or other parts of the property that are open to visitors); *Kentucky v. King*, 563 U.S. 452, 131 S. Ct. 1849 (2011).

formed officers, by physically maneuvering the individual in a particular direction, or by the intimidating use of enforcement canines;

(7) that consent was obtained only after the investigating officer retained possession of the consenting party's identification or plane, train or bus ticket;

(8) that consent was obtained only after an officer informed the consenting party that if he were innocent, he would cooperate with the police; or

(9) that the consent was given by a person already in custody or placed under arrest, and (i) the arrest occurred late at night, (ii) the arrest was made with a display of weaponry, or (iii) the arrest was made by a forcible entry or by use of force against the person.[12]

Those factors suggesting that the consent was voluntarily given include:

(1) that the consenting party was not under arrest or in custody at the time the consent was given;

(2) that (if in custody) the consenting party's custodial status was voluntary;

(3) that consent was given where the consenting party had reason to believe that the police would find no contraband;

(4) that the consenting party was aware of his constitutional right to refuse consent;

(5) that the consenting party was informed by the police prior to the request for consent of what exactly they were looking for;

---

[12] *See generally* 4 Wayne R. LaFave, *Search and Seizure: A Treatise on the Fourth Amendment*, §8.2(b) (5th ed. 2012; 2017–2018 pocket part).

(6) that the consenting party signed a "consent-to-search" form prior to the search;

(7) that the consenting party admitted his guilt before giving consent;

(8) that the consenting party affirmatively assisted the police in conducting the search;

(9) that the consenting party used his own key to provide the police with access to the area to be searched;

(10) that the consenting party had a cooperative posture throughout the encounter;

(11) that the consenting party was not in any way restrained by the police;

(12) that the consenting party knew the officers conducting the search;

(13) that the consenting party was educated or intelligent; and

(14) that the consenting party was no stranger to the criminal justice system.[13]

Note that if, in an attempt to gain consent to search a residence, officers mislead a person by saying or implying they have a warrant and will search anyway, when in reality they do not, any permission given is invalid.[14] However, the threat to obtain a warrant, while

---

[13] *See generally* 4 Wayne R. LaFave, *Search and Seizure: A Treatise on the Fourth Amendment*, §8.2(b) (5th ed. 2012; 2017–2018 pocket part); *see also United States v. Mendenhall*, 446 U.S. 544, 555-57, 100 S. Ct. 1870, 1877-78 (1980); *United States v. Watson*, 423 U.S. 411, 424, 96 S. Ct. 820, 828 (1976); *United States v. Carter*, 854 F.2d 1102, 1106 (8th Cir. 1988); *United States v. Galberth*, 846 F.2d 983 (5th Cir. 1988); *United States v. Morrow*, 731 F.2d 233, 236 (4th Cir. 1984); *United States v. Ruigomez*, 702 F.2d 61, 65 (5th Cir. 1983); *United States v. Robinson*, 690 F.2d 869, 875 (11th Cir. 1982).

[14] *Bumper v. North Carolina*, 391 U.S. 543 (1968); see also 4 Wayne R. LaFave, *Search and Seizure: A Treatise on the Fourth Amendment*, §8.2(c) (5th ed. 2012; 2017–2018 pocket part).

bearing on the voluntariness of consent, is not treated the same. Stating that a warrant can and will be obtained, if police in fact have the requisite grounds, will not automatically vitiate an ensuing consent.

§8.4. Express or Implied Consent

A consent sufficient to avoid the necessity of a warrant may be expressed or implied from the circumstances surrounding the police-citizen encounter. In fact, an *implied* consent has been held to be as effective as any express consent to search. A consent may be "implied" when it is found to exist merely because of the person's particular responses to police inquiry or the person's conduct in engaging in a certain activity.[15] Thus, an implied voluntary consent may be found where the defendant has initiated police contact and has adopted a cooperative posture in the mistaken belief that he could thereby divert or prevent police suspicion of him.

§8.5. Common Authority

A valid consent may also be obtained from one other than the accused, i.e., from a third party, so long as the consenting third party has the authority to bind the accused. In these circumstances, the inquiry whether a third-party consent is constitutionally valid focuses on whether the consenting third party possesses *common authority* over or other sufficient relationship to the premises or effects sought to be inspected.[16] The concept of third-party consent rests not upon the law of property, however, but upon the "mutual use of the property by persons generally having joint access or control for most purposes, so that it is reasonable to recognize that any of the cohabitants has the right to permit the inspection in his own right and that others have assumed the risk that one of their

---

[15] *See, e.g., United States v. Price,* 599 F.2d 494 (2d Cir. 1979) (valid search where defendant told police he did not care if they searched bag because it was not his and he had picked it up by mistake); see also *North Carolina v. Butler,* 441 U.S. 369, 375-76, 99 S. Ct. 1755, 1758-59 (1979) (an express waiver is not invariably necessary to support a finding that the defendant waived his rights).

[16] *Matlock v. United States,* 415 U.S. 164, 169-172, 94 S. Ct. 988, 993 (1974).

number might permit the common area to be searched."[17] Naturally, the prosecution must also demonstrate that the third-party consent was given freely and voluntarily.

Even where the party granting permission does not in fact have legally sufficient control over the premises, the consent may nonetheless be valid under the Fourth Amendment if the officer reasonably believes that the party had common control.[18] This is the rule for "apparent authority."

§8.6. Co-occupants

When one co-occupant of a residence consents to a search, but another co-occupant is also physically present and expressly objects to the search, then any subsequent search and seizure is unreasonable and invalid as to the objecting party. Thus, in *Georgia v. Randolph*,[19] defendant's wife called police regarding a domestic disturbance. When officers arrived, defendant was not home, but his wife alleged that he had a cocaine habit, and that he had drug paraphernalia in the house. While officers were speaking with defendant's wife, defendant returned home. He denied he had a drug habit, but also refused to consent to a search of the residence. Undeterred, the officer who asked defendant for consent then turned to defendant's wife and asked her; she readily agreed to let him search, leading the officer to a bedroom, where the officer saw a section of a drinking straw covered with a powdery residue. Because defendant had been present at the start of the search and objected to it, the contraband the officer observed could not be used against him.[20] The rule in *Randolph* does not apply, however, if the objecting occupant is not physically present at the residence—this is true even if police are the reason for the occupant's absence (i.e., if the occupant was lawfully detained or arrested prior to the request for consent to search being made).[21]

---

[17] *Id.* at 169-172, 94 S. Ct. at 993.
[18] *Illinois v. Rodriguez*, 497 U.S. 177, 110 S. Ct. 2793 (1990).
[19] *Georgia v. Randolph*, 547 U.S. 103, 120, 126 S. Ct. 1515, 1527 (2006).
[20] *Id.* at 120, 126 S. Ct. at 1527.
[21] *See Fernandez v. California*, 571 U.S. ___, 134 S. Ct. 1126 (2014).

Although a police officer may not remove someone from the premises for the purpose of preventing an objection, the officer is not required to locate an absent person to obtain the person's consent.[22]

§8.7. The Scope of the Consent

The search must be limited to those areas to which the defendant actually or implicitly gives permission to search. The scope of the search is generally determined with reference to that which the officer is seeking, i.e., to areas or containers where the stated subject of the search could be located.[23] For example, in *Florida v. Jimeno*,[24] the United States Supreme Court approved the search of a paper bag, found on the floor of a car, for narcotics, after the defendant had given consent to a general search of his car. The Court concluded that, based on these facts, it was reasonable for the searching officer to believe the scope of the consent given permitted him to open the bag. The defendant knew the purpose of the search was to look for drugs, and it was objectively reasonable to assume drugs could be found there.

Consent to search may be limited in scope, and consent may be revoked. Any evidence obtained up to the time wherein the suspect revoked his consent is admissible. Once the suspect revokes his consent to search, however, the police must stop the search, unless some other basis justifies a continuation. If the police, for example, find illegal drugs during a consent search, they may arrest the suspect. They may then conduct a search incident to arrest, even if the suspect withdraws his consent to search after the discovery of illegal drugs. Because the illegal drugs were discovered before the withdrawal of the consent, they would be admissible. The continued search after the withdrawal of consent would be permitted because it would be based on a search incident to arrest rather than consent.

---

[22] *Georgia v. Randolph*, 547 U.S. 103, 121-122, 126 S. Ct. 1515, 1527 (2006).
[23] *State v. Marshall*, 791 P.2d 880 (Utah Ct. App. 1990).
[24] *Florida v. Jimeno*, 500 U.S. 248, 111 S. Ct. 1801 (1991).

§8.8. Obtaining Consent in Special Cases

(a) *Obtaining consent from a minor.* Whether a minor possesses the authority to give law enforcement officers consent to search depends on the minor's age, intelligence, maturity, and education level.

(b) *Obtaining consent from the elderly.* To determine whether the elderly may provide a "knowing and intelligent" consent depends on a number of factors, including the person's "capacity to consent." For example, in United States v. Richards,[25] officers attempted to execute an arrest warrant at a particular residence in Fort Wayne, Indiana. Although the person named in the warrant was not present, there were others in the house, one of whom, a Mr. Edward Rawls, gave the officers consent to search. During the interaction, an officer read Rawls his *Miranda* rights. Rawls was never handcuffed or detained. The officer "gave Rawls time to read the consent form on his own and read portions of the form aloud to Rawls as well. [The officer] informed Rawls of his right to refuse consent and his right to seek legal counsel. Rawls told the officers that he understood his rights and willingly signed the consent form on the officers' first request to do so."[26]

"Throughout their interaction with Rawls, the officers did not notice anything unusual about his behavior. Officer Ealing was a member of the Fort Wayne Crisis Intervention Team and had received specialized training on how to identify people who suffer from mental illnesses. Neither officer observed signs that Rawls was experiencing any kind of dementia or confusion. Additionally, neither officer noticed any slurred speech, detected the smell of alcohol on Rawls' breath or discerned an indication that Rawls was intoxicated."[27]

In his appeal, defendant argued that Rawls did not have the requisite mental capacity to freely and voluntarily consent. Defendant contended that Rawls was incapable of consenting to the officers' search "because his advanced age of eighty-six years left

---

[25] 741 F.3d 843 (7th Cir. 2014).
[26] *Id.* at 846.
[27] *Id.* at 846-47.

Obtaining Consent to Search 221

him a confused old man who was out of touch with reality."[28] The court disagreed. Considering the information known to the officers when they arrived at Rawls' house on the day in question, the court said:

> It was readily apparent to the officers that Rawls was an older gentleman because he clearly had difficulty walking. However, nothing occurred to put the officers on notice that Rawls lacked the intelligence or the capacity to voluntarily consent to the search of his home. When Officers Ealing and Llewellyn first talked to Rawls, Rawls confirmed that he was the homeowner and invited the officers to search for Wilson [the person named in the arrest warrant]. Rawls was accompanied by two other men during this conversation, and neither of them expressed any concerns about Rawls' mental condition. Officer Ealing testified that he did not observe any signs of dementia during his interaction with Rawls. Officer Llewellyn testified that he did not notice any signs that Rawls suffered from mental problems either. Rawls did not make any inappropriate comments or act in a way that would lead the officers to believe he was confused, delusional, or unable to consent. We find nothing that would have put a reasonable officer on notice that Rawls' mental state was so impaired that he could not provide voluntary consent to the impending warrantless search.[29]

According to the court, "a person's mental capacity is only one factor in determining whether someone's consent was voluntary."[30] Said the court: "[A] person is not precluded from consenting to a warrantless search simply because he or she suffers from a mental disease."[31] In this case, there was "no evidence that Rawls suffered from a diagnosed mental disability or that officers had any reason to believe that he could not consent to the search of his home. Three officers testified about their interactions with Rawls; each concluded that Rawls appeared to understand his rights and be free of mental defects. Officer Ealing was specially trained to recognize symptoms of mental illness, and he testified that Rawls appeared to have 'all his

---

[28] *Id.* at 847.
[29] *Id.* at 848.
[30] *Id.* at 849.
[31] *Id.*

mental faculties about him.' Without evidence of aberrant behavior from Rawls" on the day in question, the court concluded that "Rawls was capable of voluntarily consenting to the officers' search."[32]

(c) *Obtaining consent from the injured, intoxicated, drugged or those in ill health.* Similar to the analysis in confession law, persons who are in pain, intoxicated or on drugs may not be able to give a voluntary, knowing, and intelligent consent to search. As in confession law, the prosecution has the burden of showing by a preponderance of the evidence that the consent procedure was proper.[33]

(d) *Obtaining consent from persons with diminished capacity.* The courts have held that "the mental capacity of the person giving consent is only one factor in evaluating his capacity to give voluntary consent."[34] Thus, "it should not be assumed . . . that anyone suffering from some type of mental disease or defect is inevitably incapable of giving a voluntary consent to a search."[35]

---

[32] *Id.*

[33] *See Colorado v. Connelly,* 479 U.S. 157, 166, 107 S. Ct. 515 (1986) (In the context of determining the voluntariness of a confession where defendant suffered from a psychosis that interfered with his ability to make free and rational choices and exclusively relied on his mental condition, the Supreme Court stated, "Only if we were to establish a brand new constitutional right-the right of a criminal defendant to confess to his crime only when totally rational and properly motivated-could [defendant's] present claim be sustained."). *See also United States v. Montgomery,* 621 F.3d at 572, 573 (rejecting "a per se rule that medication (or intoxication) necessarily defeats an individual's capacity to consent," the Sixth Circuit compared the Fifth Amendment waiver and Fourth Amendment consent-to-search inquiries, and noted, that "the 'knowing and intelligent' prong of the *Miranda* waiver inquiry is more protective of individual liberty than the consent-to-search doctrine because it requires a 'full awareness of both the nature of the right being abandoned and the consequences of the decision to abandon it,' namely, a *Miranda* warning, something not required in Fourth Amendment consent cases.") (citations omitted)).

[34] *United States v. Grap,* 403 F.3d 439, 445 (7th Cir. 2005).

[35] 4 Wayne R. LaFave, *Search and Seizure: A Treatise on the Fourth Amendment,* 8.2(e) (5th ed. 2012); see also *United States v. Ingram,* No. 3:10-cr-00069, 2010 U.S. Dist. LEXIS 139041, 2010 WL 5441671, at *11-12 (W.D.N.C. Dec. 28, 2010) (concluding that although the consenter suffered from dementia, the officer's conclusion of voluntariness was reasonable in light of the consenter's behavior as presented to the officer); *Brewster v. New York,* No. 08-CV-4653, 2010 U.S. Dist. LEXIS 887, 2010 WL 92884, at *7 (E.D.N.Y. Jan. 6, 2010) (rejecting defendant's claim that he was incapable of giving consent due to a mental disease or defect, the court explained that the relevant question is not whether defendant in fact suffered from a mental disease or defect at the time he consented to the search, rather the question is an objective one-whether under the totality of the circumstances was the consent voluntary or involuntary? The court concluded,

"Modern medicine allows those suffering from even severe forms of mental illness ... to control their conditions through medication."[36]

For example, in *United States v. Grap*,[37] defendant Daniel Grap was charged with various offenses related to the possession of stolen firearms. During the investigation, Detective Gallagher obtained consent to search from defendant's mother. At defendant's home, Gallagher informed Mrs. Grap that his visit concerned stolen property that he believed to be in her garage and asked for her permission to search that building. Mrs. Grap then asked Detective Gallagher if he was looking for guns. The detective had not yet disclosed to Mrs. Grap the nature of the stolen property for which he was searching. Detective Gallagher then produced a written consent form, read it aloud to Mrs. Grap, and handed it to her. After Mrs. Grap reviewed and signed the form, Detective Gallagher also signed it. Mrs. Grap asked no further questions about the form and appeared to understand it.

Thereafter, Mrs. Grap opened the detached garage door with a garage door opener, and Detective Gallagher entered and found three rifles. He then carried these rifles out to his police vehicle and placed them on the hood of his car. At this point, Mrs. Grap came back outside and asked Detective Gallagher what he was going to do with the guns. When Detective Gallagher informed her that he believed the guns were stolen, and that he would be taking them with him, Mrs. Grap stated that the guns might belong to her husband. Detective Gallagher asked Mrs. Grap if her husband kept his guns in the garage; she replied that he usually kept them in a closet in the house, prompting Detective Gallagher to request that she check to make sure her husband's guns were still there. Mrs. Grap reentered her house and emerged a moment later to inform Detective Gallagher that her husband's guns were still in the closet. Detective Gallagher then told Mrs. Grap that he would take the guns found in the garage and provided her with a handwritten receipt

---

"There is nothing in the record to suggest that petitioner was not lucid and cooperative while dealing with police. Nor were there signs in the record that petitioner was suffering from delusional symptoms or any other serious impairment that would indicate to a reasonable officer that the consent was not voluntary.").

[36] *United States v. Grap*, 403 F.3d 439, 445 (7th Cir. 2005).
[37] 403 F.3d 439 (7th Cir. 2005).

listing the descriptions of the guns and their serial numbers. Mrs. Grap did not ask any questions about the receipt, and both she and Detective Gallagher signed it.

According to Detective Gallagher, Mrs. Grap appeared to understand everything he had said that day and did not seem confused; thus, at no time did he believe that she lacked the capacity to consent to the warrantless search of her garage.[38]

At the hearing on defendant's motion to suppress evidence, it was argued that Mrs. Grap could not provide a voluntary and knowing consent. Mr. Grap and a psychiatrist testified that she was mentally ill and that "her psychosis" rendered her unable to provide a valid consent. Richard Grap testified that his wife had suffered from mental illness for at least ten years, and had refused to take her medication in the time period between January and May of the relevant year. "Dr. Jack Rodriguez, Mrs. Grap's psychiatrist, testified that she had been hospitalized for a delusional disorder that impaired her ability to make rational decisions, and that she refused to take her medication when she was not in the hospital, causing her to become increasingly delusional and out of touch. According to Dr. Rodriguez, at times Mrs. Grap could appear to be fairly lucid, but might nonetheless be in a delusional state."[39]

The trial court ruled that Mrs. Grap possessed the mental capacity to make a rational decision as to whether to give or withhold her consent to the warrantless search, and denied Grap's motion to suppress physical evidence. The Court of Appeals agreed. In deciding this case, the Court explained that whether a consent to search is "voluntary" is dependent upon the totality of the circumstances.

Among the factors that aid in determining whether consent was freely given are the age, education, and intelligence and (applicable here) mental health and capability of the person giving consent; whether the person giving consent did so immediately or only after repeated requests by the police; whether physical coercion was used

---

[38] *Id.* at 441.
[39] *Id.* at 441-442.

to obtain consent; and whether the person giving consent was in custody .... [40]

[W]e find that Detective Gallagher properly obtained Mrs. Grap's voluntary consent to search the Grap premises. [H]e informed Mrs. Grap that he believed that there was stolen property in her garage, asked her permission to search and then produced a consent form and read it aloud to Mrs. Grap ....

The evidence also persuades us that, despite her mental infirmities, Mrs. Grap freely and voluntarily consented to Detective Gallagher's search, and that she was aware of all the relevant circumstances of the search and seizure of the stolen firearms. There is no allegation that Mrs. Grap lacked the authority to give consent to the warrantless search. And however potentially serious the effects of her psychosis, Mrs. Grap's behavior did not indicate that she lacked the requisite mental capacity to consent. When Detective Gallagher informed her of his belief that stolen property was in her garage without disclosing the nature of the property, Mrs. Grap asked him whether he was searching for guns. Mrs. Grap also signed both the consent form and the receipt, and opened the door of the garage with a garage door opener. Once Detective Gallagher had recovered the rifles, Mrs. Grap mentioned that the guns might belong to her husband, and had the good sense to inform Detective Gallagher that her husband kept his guns in their bedroom and, after checking, to confirm that her husband's guns were indeed in this location. This behavior would clearly indicate to a reasonable observer that Mrs. Grap sufficiently understood the consequences of her consent. And reasonableness is the touchstone of validity of third-party consent to a search.[41]

* * * *

Here, an [in depth analysis of whether] Mrs. Grap's mental condition, as determined by psychiatric testimony, prevented her from having the requisite mental capacity to voluntarily consent to a warrantless search might be of academic interest, but it has little to

---

[40] *Id.* at 443.
[41] *Id.* at 443-444 (citing *Illinois v. Rodriguez,* 497 U.S. 177, 182, 110 S.Ct. 2793, 2798 (1990)).

do with regulating police conduct. The proper inquiry here focuses on the objective facts, as presented to a reasonable inquirer, that would reasonably put him or her on notice that a voluntary consent could not be given.

[M]ental capacity of the person giving consent is only one factor in evaluating his capacity to give voluntary consent. And [m]odern medicine allows those suffering from even severe forms of mental illness, including, apparently, Mrs. Grap, to control their conditions through medication. Though Mrs. Grap has a history of refusing to take prescribed medication, her behavior provides no indication that she was suffering from delusional symptoms, or that she was "out of touch" with reality. On the contrary, she acted as if she were profoundly aware of events as they unfolded.

Our approach to the question of mental capacity to consent to a search may be analogized to the issue of apparent authority addressed in *Illinois v. Rodriguez*. That case holds that a person with apparent authority (that is, a person having the indicia of agency as opposed to one actually authorized) may validly consent to a search. "Even if [the purported agent] did not in fact have authority to give consent, it suffices to validate the entry that the law enforcement officers reasonably believed she did."[42]

Similarly, in *United States v. Strache*,[43] the defendant, who was allegedly mentally ill and suicidal at the time of the search, sought to suppress evidence of explosives that police had uncovered in a warrantless search of his bedroom by claiming that his mental condition rendered him incapable of giving free and voluntary consent. The court disagreed, finding that the defendant's consent was voluntary based on the police officers' testimony that the defendant was clear and lucid and had behaved in a relaxed and cooperative manner. In Strache, the impressions presented to the officers were undeniably relevant and, in fact, determinative in the court's analysis of whether the consent was voluntary under the totality of the circumstances. The court held that the officers'

---

[42] *Id.* at 444.
[43] 202 F.3d 980, 985 (7th Cir. 2000).

conclusions of voluntariness were reasonable in light of the defendant's behavior, as presented to the officers.[44]

---

[44] *But see United States v. Elrod,* 441 F.2d 353, 355 (5th Cir. 1971), where the Fifth Circuit suppressed physical evidence of a bank robbery that police officers had uncovered in a warrantless search of a hotel room that was occupied by the defendant and codefendant, finding that the codefendant, who suffered from schizophrenia, lacked mental capacity when he consented to the warrantless search. The Fifth Circuit explained its holding by asserting that, "no matter how genuine the belief of the officers is that the consentor is apparently of sound mind, and deliberately acting, the search depending on his consent fails if it is judicially determined that he lacked mental capacity." 441 F.2d at 355. However, the Fifth Circuit also noted that the "question was one of mental awareness so that the act of consent was the consensual act of one who knew what he was doing and had a reasonable appreciation of the nature and significance of his actions." *Id.* at 355.

The critical difference between the approaches to voluntary consent in Strache and Elrod stems from the weight to be accorded the evidence presented to a reasonable officer asking for consent as opposed to some other facts, unknown to the officer, but later argued to the reviewing court. There may be an inference in Elrod that this after-presented evidence is relevant, but in the Strache approach, it would be relevant only to impeach the credibility of the officer or to shed any light on what was reasonably apparent to him when he obtained the consent. The standard of what is reasonably apparent to a reasonable inquiring officer, with its emphasis on the deterrence rationale of the exclusionary rule, has been held to be the correct approach by most courts. Clearly, officers should not be deterred by circumstances that are unknown to them, like the psychiatric history of the person consenting to a search. *See United States v. Merritt,* 361 F.3d 1005, 1009 (7th Cir. 2004) (reversed on other grounds) (quoting *United States v. Calandra,* 414 U.S. 338, 348, 94 S. Ct. 613 (1974)).

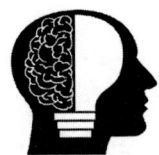

KEY POINTS

- A "consent to search" procedure is treated by the courts as a recognized exception to the written warrant requirement.

- To be valid, a consent must be voluntary, knowing, and intelligent.

- When consent is voluntary, it is freely and intelligently given, uncontaminated by any duress or coercion, actual or implied.

- In all cases, the question whether a consent to a search was in fact voluntary or was the product of duress or coercion, express or implied, is a question of fact to be determined from the "totality of the circumstances."

- The prosecution has the burden of proof to show that the consent to search was freely and voluntarily given.

- Third-party consents are valid, so long as the consenting third party possesses common authority over or other sufficient relationship to the premises or effects sought to be inspected.

- The concept of third-party consent rests not on the law of property, however, but on the mutual use of the property by persons generally having joint access or control for most purposes.

KEY POINTS (Continued)

- When one co-occupant of a residence consents to a search, but another co-occupant is also physically present and expressly objects to the search, then any subsequent search and seizure is unreasonable and invalid as to the objecting party.

- Whether a minor possesses the authority to give law enforcement officers consent to search depends on the minor's age, intelligence, maturity, and education.

- To determine whether the elderly may provide a "knowing and intelligent" consent depends on a number of factors, including the person's "capacity to consent."

- Similar to the analysis in confession law, persons who are in pain, intoxicated or on drugs may not be able to give a voluntary, knowing, and intelligent consent to search; it will depend on the totality of the circumstances.

- The courts have held that the mental capacity of the person giving consent is only one factor in evaluating his capacity to give voluntary consent.

- It should not be assumed that anyone suffering from some type of mental disease or defect is inevitably incapable of giving a voluntary consent to a search. Modern medicine allows those suffering from even severe forms of mental illness to control their conditions through medication.

Chapter Nine
REPORT WRITING IN SPECIAL CASES

§9.1. Introduction

When responding to incidents involving persons with special needs, one of the most important responsibilities of the law enforcement officer or other first responder is report writing—the proper documentation of what was seen, heard and accomplished. Too often, unfortunately, insufficient attention is devoted to critical observations at the time of response. Proper attention, however, could save the first responder from subsequent second guessing by superiors, defense attorneys and the courts.

The incident reports prepared by law enforcement officers and other first responders often become part of an official record, which documents the history of an emergency or other type of response, a critical incident, event or crime. Nearly every dispatched service a first responder performs, each crime and accident scene a law enforcement officer investigates, and any other criminal justice operation requiring that a record be made for future reference, calls for an accurately worded entry in a log or a detailed chronicle of information, commonly known as the "officer's official report." Although the length of these reports may vary, each has one common purpose: to communicate information in an accurate, understandable and complete manner.

To be effective, formal reports should always be written with the intended audience in mind, and with an eye toward sufficiently documenting the need for certain actions, immediately taken and subsequently taken. This latter aspect is important when an officer needs to take a certain approach with a person with special needs. In this regard, it is important to recognize that such reports may be viewed by supervisors, the media, social service agencies, physicians, psychiatrists and insurance companies. In the criminal justice system, an officer's report will be read and analyzed by prosecutors, defense attorneys and judges. Consequently, the quality and effectiveness of an officer's report can help to assist the person with special needs, convict the guilty and respect the rights of crime victims.

§9.2. Proper Documentation

Even if an officer is simply providing transportation for a person in the officer's patrol car, the action should be documented, albeit briefly in the officer's patrol log. Naturally, the more involved the response, the more involved the reporting. Even if you believe the action does not constitute "official action," if it affects the life, liberty or property of another person in any significant way, document your actions and observations. It is all too easy, at a later date, to connect any of your actions—official or other—to your authoritative position as a public safety officer. Proper documentation is your best protection.

§9.3. Maintaining a Proper Frame of Reference

To maintain a proper frame of reference, you must not only assess an event from your perspective but must also determine how something may be perceived by others. View your writing and your overall report from the eyes of your audience, be it a supervisor, physician, prosecutor, district attorney, judge or defense attorney. Does your documentation support why you took a certain course of action? Can a lack of documentation be used against you?

For example, in a previous chapter, we discussed the case of *United States v. Richards*,[1] where officers obtained consent to search from a Mr. Edward Rawls, the 86-year-old homeowner. During the consent-search procedure, Rawls was never handcuffed or detained. The officers read him his rights, and they "gave Rawls time to read the consent form on his own and read portions of the form aloud to Rawls as well. [The officer] informed Rawls of his right to refuse consent and his right to seek legal counsel. Rawls told the officers that he understood his rights and willingly signed the consent form

---

[1] 741 F.3d 843 (7th Cir. 2014).

on the officers' first request to do so."[2] This is the type of interaction that must be meticulously documented. The officers are obtaining consent to search from an 86-year-old. They should expect a legal challenge down the road.

"Throughout their interaction with Rawls, the officers did not notice anything unusual about his behavior. Officer Ealing was a member of the Fort Wayne Crisis Intervention Team and had received specialized training on how to identify people who suffer from mental illnesses. Neither officer observed signs that Rawls was experiencing any kind of dementia or confusion. Additionally, neither officer noticed any slurred speech, detected the smell of alcohol on Rawls' breath or discerned an indication that Rawls was intoxicated."[3] These critical observations must be documented in the officer's formal report.

Because the officers properly documented the incident and were able to comprehensively testify as to the totality of the circumstances surrounding the consent process, the court was quick to reject the defendant's argument on appeal that Rawls did not have the mental capacity to freely and voluntarily consent "because his advanced age of eighty-six years left him a confused old man who was out of touch with reality."[4] Based on the officer's report and testimony, the court pointed out that there was nothing that occurred "to put the officers on notice that Rawls lacked the intelligence or the capacity to voluntarily consent to the search of his home." Officer Ealing properly documented and testified that he did not observe any signs of dementia during his interaction with Rawls, and Officer Llewellyn testified that he did not notice any signs that Rawls suffered from any sort of mental problems. "Rawls did not make any inappropriate comments or act in a way that would lead the officers to believe he was confused, delusional, or unable to consent."[5] Consequently, the officers' proper documentation saved the constitutionality of the consent-search procedure.

---

[2] *Id.* at 846.
[3] *Id.* at 846–47.
[4] *Id.* at 847.
[5] *Id.* at 848.

§9.4. Ensure Proper Tone

It is always important to remember who will be reading your report—your audience. The "who's my audience" perspective ensures proper tone. In writing, tone refers to the writer's attitude toward the subject of the communication and the reader. The overall tone of the written report can directly impact how the reader will interpret what is said.

For example, when describing a particular person, writing that the person was "dirty," strikes an improper tone. It is also imprecise. What does the term "dirty" mean? Does it mean that the person is involved in criminal activity? Does it mean that the person is in possession of illegal narcotics? Or does it mean that the person has black and brown dirt on his arms and clothing and smells like he or she has not bathed in quite a while?

Reporting that the person was "crazy" or "off the wall" does not help describe what is actually being observed. Instead, supply the actual detail of what the person was doing.

> *Example:*
>
> A frantic female clerk calls 911 reporting a sexual predator in the convenience store. You are dispatched to the call. On arrival, you observe an elderly man wearing sneakers, underwear and a jacket walking around the store. You hear him say, "Do you know where I live?, Can you take me home?" The man begins to cry. Would you describe this man as "crazy" or "off the wall"? Is this person a criminal? He was not harming anyone and was distraught. Due to his advanced age, a safe assumption may be that he has dementia and wandered away from home. A detailed description of this event describes a man in need of assistance. The store clerk was frantic because of this situation, all she saw was someone in undergarments acting in an unusual manner. She called 911. In her mind it translated to "sexual predator"—that's how

Report Writing in Special Cases   235

> she interpreted the situation. She saw only the underwear and the behavior. Her description had the officers prepared for an entirely different response. The man was not a sexual predator but an elderly man with dementia who needed assistance.

Sometimes the individual calling in to 911 improperly describes the situation. This can occur because of fear, anxiety, and lack of training. They are upset and see the circumstance through their own filter. Things are not always as described by the bystander.

A detailed report would explain:

1) *What and Where:* What was reported in the 911 call and where it took place. This helps to set the tone and describe what you were anticipating.

2) *The circumstances:* Accurately describe what you observe; details are important here. You are painting a picture with words to represent the event. Detailed descriptions will help you reconstruct the events at a later time. Your description should depict the circumstances so accurately that anyone reading your report will be able to "see" in their mind's eye what occurred; whether it's you, your supervisor, or an attorney. Imagine that you are in court on the witness stand. When you are asked a question you simply refer to your report. It's that simple. Put the time into writing an effective descriptive report. That report can and will protect and defend your actions later.

3) *The Actions Taken:* Describe what you did, describe your response.

4) *The Resolution:* How was the call resolved.

5) *The Takeaway:* You are describing a scene that has a *beginning* (the what and where), a *middle* (the circumstances and the actions taken), and an *end* (the resolution, how the call was resolved).

> *Example:*
>
> In the following example, the officer describes the event in his report.
>
> > *I arrived at the scene and observed someone on the ground having some kind of "fit." A few people were around, watching. There was a person who looked weird and dirty standing over the guy; he wouldn't answer me or follow my directions. He was so "off the wall," that I had to handcuff him to get him under control. I put him in my squad car because he was crying and screaming. I left him there and called for an ambulance for the other guy.*

Granted, the description above is an extreme example of improper report writing. The officer involved may have acted in a more professional manner in the actual circumstance, but his report does not reflect it. He clearly was dealing with individuals with special needs without proper training. The example demonstrates a lack of training, sensitivity and understanding of the proper terminology. Referring to an individual as having a "fit" is improper. Using terms that are outdated, offensive and negative demonstrates a lack of training and compassion. Moreover, those terms do not effectively describe the circumstances.

A better way to handle the event and effectively describe the actions taken would be:

> *When I arrived at the scene I observed a man in his twenties lying on the ground. He appeared to be convulsing, perhaps having a serious seizure. I immediately called for an ambulance. There were three people around the person. One of the individuals was crying, and pulling at his clothes and hair. His jacket was torn and soiled. He appeared to be in his twenties. I asked everyone to step back and give the person on the ground some room. I asked everyone to stay so I could determine what occurred. I cleared the area around the person,*

Report Writing in Special Cases

> *which was scattered with debris, so the victim could not injure himself. The individual who was crying was still standing very close and did not respond to my request to move back. I repeated my request a second time, but there was no response. I moved closer; as I did, he began to rock back and forth. I quickly backed up and he stopped rocking. I realized that I was dealing with a person with special needs. I said, "My name is Officer Phillips, I am here to help. An ambulance is on the way. Do you understand?" The person still did not look at me but shook his head yes. "Good, I'm glad you understand. I see that you have been crying, are you hurt?" The individual shook his head no. "I'm glad you are OK." The ambulance arrived and began to care for the individual. I was then able to question the others at the scene.*

Ensuring proper tone requires that you think before you write. Ambiguous, vague or confused reporting results from a failure to think through the facts and circumstances, which will ultimately make up the body or narrative of the report. The best descriptions are detailed and objective. Writing that the person was "dirty," or "crazy," or "off the wall" is not sufficiently descriptive to alert the reader as to what actually was observed and what truly occurred.

Think through each portion of your report from beginning to end; then write. This will not only provide the clarity and coherence so necessary for effective official reporting, but it may also protect you should your conduct be called into question at some point in the future. Further, it will eliminate the need for future translation, particularly during an official court proceeding.

§9.5. Field Notes

When responding to incidents involving persons with special needs, your field notes may serve as your first-responder's official memory. Whether taken in an actual notebook, iPad, audio recorder or similar device, field notes are a critical part of the process. Indeed, studies have shown that the mere act of writing something down or recording it in a device will impress it more deeply in your memory. Don't rely on your ability to remember each particular fact or event. Chances are, you will inevitably forget something important.

Properly taken field notes will provide you with a shorthand or abbreviated record (whether written or audio recorded) of what was seen, said or done. If taken properly, field notes will greatly reduce the risk of the inaccurate reporting of names; addresses; dates of birth; social security numbers; serial numbers; times; locations of evidence, witnesses, victims, or suspects; distances; and so on. Thereafter, your field notes serve as an index to your memory of the event in question, and as the basis for your formal report.

§9.6. Body-Worn Cameras

With more and more agencies utilizing body-worn cameras ("BWCs"), a more complete record of the circumstances leading up to an officer's actions, along with the actions themselves, is now available. When using a BWC, the officer must always respect the privacy interests of persons whose images and home interiors may be captured in a BWC recording. It is also important to recognize the benefits achieved by BWC evidence that might help to solve a crime and successfully prosecute an offender.

Ultimately, it is the public safety agency's decision whether to provide its officers with BWCs to deploy in the field. Their use clearly can play an important role in addressing public concerns about a law enforcement officer's use of force, particularly if it involves a shooting, as well as an officer's actions to restrain a violent or unruly suspect. The practical utility of BWCs lies not only in their ability to record objectively the circumstances of an officer–civilian confrontation, but also in their capacity to discourage both officers and civilians from engaging in inappropriate conduct. These devices also can serve to discourage both law enforcement and civilian witnesses from providing false information about the circumstances of the encounter; a BWC recording not only can vindicate an officer who is falsely accused of misconduct, and do so

Report Writing in Special Cases

very quickly, but also will discourage a person from making false allegations against the officer in the first place.[6]

BWC recordings may also be used for the more routine documentation of visual and aural evidence learned in the course of conducting police investigations. Not only will BWC recordings preserve accurate visual depictions of physical evidence, such as weapons and illicit drugs and paraphernalia, but also will document where and how physical evidence was found. BWCs also will record the physical appearance of suspects, witnesses, crime victims, and individuals with special needs. The devices help preserve evidence of any apparent injuries, infirmities, illnesses, maladies, disorders, afflictions (not the most euphemistic version of this term), frailties and other special problems. The audio portion of BWC recordings, meanwhile, will document witness and suspect statements, preserving not only the substantive content of those statements, but also showing whether officers had complied with *Miranda* and other legal requirements.[7]

"Although BWCs record events accurately and objectively, they do not replace the need for complete and accurate police reports and testimony. The fact that a BWC is not activated to record an encounter or event does not, of course, preclude an officer from testifying as to the circumstances of the encounter or event, or affect the admissibility of evidence. Nor does it suggest that the officer's written report or testimony is inaccurate or incomplete. However, a BWC recording can supplement and corroborate the accuracy of written reports and testimony, which is one of the significant benefits of deploying these devices."[8] Note also that BWCs do not capture every detail; for instance, if the event takes place at night certain details may not be obvious. If the person has dilated eyes, smells of gasoline, or has white powder under his or her nose and is mildly shaking, a BWC may not convey these details. It is up to you to put it in your report.

---

[6] *New Jersey Attorney General Directive No. 2015-1 Regarding Police Body Worn Cameras (BWCs) and Stored BWC Recordings,* July 28, 2015, at p. 3: http://www.nj.gov/lps/dcj/agguide/directives/2015-1_BWC.pdf

[7] *Id.*

[8] *Id.*

§9.7. Report Writing Checklist

_____ I. WHO
  A. Who is reporting?
  B. Who called the police?
  C. Who is (are) the victim(s)? Complainant(s)? Witness(es)?
  D. Who discovered the event (if different from complainant)?
  E. Who is (are) the suspect(s)?
  F. Who has been arrested?
  G. Who is (are) the arresting officer(s)?

_____ II. WHAT
  A. Type of incident
  B. If of a criminal nature:
     1. Statutory violation
     2. Prohibited conduct
  C. If other than criminal
     1. Circumstances
     2. Persons involved; comments; statements
     3. Special circumstances

_____ III. WHERE
  A. Where did the incident occur?
  B. Where was (were) the victim(s) found?
  C. Where was (were) the suspect(s) found?
  D. Where was (were) the witness(es) situated in relation to the event?
  E. Where did the arrest(s) take place?
  F. Where was any property or evidence found?

_____ IV. WHEN
  A. Time and date of incident
  B. Time and date discovered; or reported
  C. Time and date victim(s) is (are) located (or identified)
  D. Time and date suspect(s) is (are) located and/or identified
  E. Time and date of any arrest
  F. Time and date of any search
  G. Time and date of *Miranda* warning administration

Report Writing in Special Cases 241

_____ V. WHY
  A. Motive
  B. Opportunity

_____ VI. HOW
  A. How was/were the crime/acts committed/performed?
  B. How did the victim(s), witness(s) look, act, respond?
  C. How did the suspect(s) look, act, respond?

_____ VII. OTHER

_____
_____
_____
_____
_____
_____
_____

§9.8. Be Sure to Include All Relevant and Necessary Facts

As long as the information has "any tendency to make the existence of any fact that is of consequence to the determination of the action more probable or less probable than it would be without the evidence,"[9] it is relevant. If you are not sure if a particular fact is a "relevant fact," that is, one which may be of consequence and make the existence of something more or less probable, include it anyway. If reasonable minds could differ over whether or not a particular fact is a relevant fact, chances are, that fact is relevant, and should be included.

Many times, the precise relevance of a specific piece of information may not be readily apparent at the time of report writing — its relevance becomes clear only later on in the investigation. This is especially true when documenting information in special needs cases.

---

[9] *Fed.R.Evid.* 401.

For example, in *State v. W.S.B.*,[10] an officer responded to a report of a person, who was described by an unidentified third-party caller as "intoxicated" in the waiting area of a train station. The officer found a person lying on the floor of the station. The officer observed the person nodding in and out of consciousness when asked questions, being unaware of his location, and displaying "pinpoint" eyes. Recognizing these characteristics were indicative of the effects of heroin use, the officer summoned an ambulance.

The EMTs transported the person, later identified as the defendant, W.S.B., from the train station to a local hospital, where he was diagnosed as having an "intentional drug overdose." Hospital staff found several used and unused bags of a heroin in defendant's backpack, which was turned over to law enforcement. Defendant moved to dismiss all charges, arguing that the state's Overdose Prevention Act protects him.

Finding those facts insufficient to determine whether the Overdoes Prevention Act applied, the court pointed out that the prosecution's case was unclear on important details. Insufficient reporting by the responding officer caused gaps in the information related to:

- the supposed hearsay report of an "intoxicated" person on the floor of the train station;

- whether any bystanders observed defendant's condition;

- what additional observations the officer made concerning defendant's actual condition, if any;

- whether defendant exhibited any signs of acute physical illness; and

- exactly why the officer called for EMT assistance and particularly whether his call was prompted by routine standard police protocols rather than an individualized assessment that defendant's condition was "acute" and required medical assistance. [11]

---

[10] 453 N.J.Super. 206, 180 A.3d 1168 (App.Div. 2018).
[11] *Id.* at 241, 180 A.3d at 1188-89.

Report Writing in Special Cases 243

Due to insufficient reporting and documentation, the court needed to remand the matter to have these topics further explored.

§9.9. Avoid Legal, Medical and Other Improper Conclusions

There is a clear-cut difference between presenting the facts and reporting an improper legal or medical conclusion.

For example:

The Facts	Improper Conclusion
I observed both suspects sitting in the rear of the vehicle, handing back and forth a plastic wrapper which contained a white powder.	I observed *suspicious behavior*.
As I attempted to place the suspect in handcuffs, another subject quickly approached, grabbed my left hand, and attempted to wrestle the handcuffs away from me.	The subject *obstructed the lawful performance of my official duty*.
I observed the individual smoking a substance that smelled like marijuana.	Based on what I saw, I had probable cause to arrest the person.
When I arrived at the scene, a man of about 80 years old was yelling at the clerk. When I approached him, he ran out of the store with a bottle of what appeared to be alcohol.	The old man with Alzheimer's was yelling at the clerk. When he saw I was an officer, he ran out of the store, stealing a bottle of liquor.
When I arrived at the scene I saw a man of about 50, standing on the porch. I approached him and observed that he appeared upset. He was shaking. He was unable to speak and was not dressed properly for the weather.	At the scene, I had to deal with a man who was obviously brain damaged and retarded. He couldn't understand simple English and was possibly deaf and dumb.
When I arrived at the scene of the accident, I observed a woman of about 30 lying on the ground. She was violently shaking and had foam coming out of her mouth.	The woman was really out of it. She was on the ground having some kind of fit. She looked retarded.

The Facts	Improper Conclusion
When I arrived at the scene of the accident, I observed a woman of about 80 years of age wearing a bathrobe and what appeared to be slippers in the driver's seat. She had driven her car into the front window of the dry cleaners. The woman stated that she did not know how it happened.	The woman, who was too old to be driving, drove her car into the store. She was out of her mind, because she told me she didn't know how it happened.

As a general rule, it is the officer's job merely to convey his or her knowledge of the facts. Once the officer relates the facts, it is the job of the court to assess those facts and then pronounce the legal conclusion. Explain what you see, do not diagnose.

§9.10. Avoid Shorthand Expressions

Public safety officials, attorneys and doctors, for that matter, love shorthand expressions. Why say a lot when you can say it all in just a couple of words? In official reporting, however, the use of shorthand expressions is inappropriate. While the use of these words may make report writing faster and easier, they are a poor replacement for necessary factual details.

The Facts	Improper Shorthand Expressions
When we arrived at the station, Mr. Jones began yelling and cursing. As soon as I opened the rear door of the patrol car, he spit in my face. He then refused to get out of the car.	When we arrived at the station, Mr. Jones became *belligerent and uncooperative.*
As I spoke with the suspect, I noticed that his hands were trembling. As he spoke, his lip quivered and his voice fluttered. Beads of sweat started to accumulate on his brow.	The suspect exhibited *extreme nervousness.*

Report Writing in Special Cases

The Facts	Improper Shorthand Expressions
The suspect then quickly reached into the inside pocket of his jacket with his left hand and attempted to grab an object of some kind.	The suspect then made a *furtive gesture*.
I immediately reached out, held the suspect's hand in place and conducted a protective frisk. When I patted the breast area of his Jacket, I touched an object that clearly felt like a gun.	After the suspect acted *suspiciously*, I *searched* him. When I felt the gun in his pocket, he started to *get violent*. I then *subdued* him by *neutralizing* his hands, and brought him in.
Immediately thereafter, the suspect quickly pulled away from my grasp, raised his hands, clenched his fists and assumed a fighting stance. As soon as he began to throw his first punch, I grabbed his arm, turned him around, applied handcuffs and informed him that he was under arrest.	The *suspect resisted arrest* and had to be subdued.

§9.11. Avoid Inappropriate Inferences

Avoid drawing inferences as to what a person may have seen, heard, felt, or believed; or what a person may have been attempting to do or not to do on a particular occasion. While it is very natural to draw such inferences from an individual's conduct, many times those inferences are wrong, or at least questionable. It is best to simply to objectively describe the individual's conduct.

The Facts	Inappropriate Inferences
As I turned the corner, I saw the subject inserting a crowbar into the side window of the American Appliance store.	As I turned the corner, I saw the subject attempting to break into the American Appliance store.

The Facts	Inappropriate Inferences
At the time, I was in full uniform. As I walked closer to where the subject stood, he quickly turned and looked directly at me. As his eyes made contact with mine, his head jerked back suddenly. He then immediately dropped the crowbar and ran.	I startled the subject as I walked closer to where he stood. As soon as he saw the police presence, he ran.
At the station, I asked the motorist for his name, address, date of birth and other biographical information. He responded with several slurred sounds, but did not answer any of the questions. There was a strong odor of an alcoholic beverage coming from him.	At the station, I asked the motorist for biographical information. He was so drunk, he could not respond.
I called out to the woman as she climbed onto the tenth-floor window ledge, but she did not answer.	I called out to the woman as she was about to commit suicide, but she couldn't hear me.

§9.12. Remain Objective

There is a definite difference between subjective and objective writing. Subjective writing expresses the writer's personal feelings or emotions, opinions, biases or prejudices, and does so generally without regard to verifiable facts and evidence. Objective writing records the facts and circumstances without reference to the writer's personal feelings of the event; without emotion; and most important, without any implications of bias or prejudice.

For example, an objective statement would be:

> A young blond female of about twenty years old was standing on the corner in a short silver skirt, a bright yellow blouse with a bare midriff and red high heels. She approached cars stopped at red lights.

Report Writing in Special Cases

A subjective statement:

> A young blond girl who looked liked a hooker, wearing sexy clothes was standing on the corner in a part of town known for prostitution. She was approaching Johns when they stopped for a red light.

As with many general rules, the rule of objectivity has a few exceptions. One exception may be found in the circumstances surrounding the drawing of your service weapon, and your justification for doing so. Part of your justification may be subjective; for example: "The subject looked like he was reaching for a weapon." This statement is important, for it shows your state of mind at the time. So long as you detail in your report the facts and circumstances that caused you to believe the subject was reaching for a weapon, the subjective statement demonstrating your state of mind at the time is proper for your formal report.

Another exception deals with the recognition of certain contraband. For example, if, during a motor vehicle stop, you notice a plastic bag containing a white powdery substance located on the vehicle's console, and a triple-beam scale resting on the back seat, you may reasonably conclude that the substance is cocaine. Under these circumstances, there is nothing wrong with including a statement in your report that, based on your training and experience, you believed the substance was cocaine (or a similar illegal substance), or that you believed the triple-beam scale was related paraphernalia. Here, it is important that the details leading up to your subjective statement must be set forth in your report.

Similarly, after detailing the obvious signs of impairment — strong odor of an alcoholic beverage on a motorist's breath, bloodshot eyes, slurred speech, poor performance on balance tests — an officer can offer an opinion that a motorist was drunk, i.e., under the influence of alcohol. Indeed, even an ordinary citizen is qualified to advance an opinion in a court proceeding that a person was intoxicated due to consumption of alcohol, because the symptoms of that condition have become "common knowledge."[12]

Certainly, there are other exceptions. "As a rule of thumb, whenever it becomes necessary to draw a conclusion in your report, or include a subjective statement demonstrating your state of mind, be sure to also detail the facts and circumstances supporting your conclusion or statement. This gives the reader the opportunity to draw his or her own conclusions, and assess whether your conclusions were reasonable."[13]

§9.13. The Use of Appropriate Words

As a general rule, choose the word that most precisely explains the event or describes the person or object under consideration. For example, when describing the events of an assault:

Bad:
The suspect punched the victim's lights out.

Better:
The suspect punched the victim in the face, causing her to lose consciousness.

Or when describing a minor motor vehicle accident involving no damage:

Bad:
Vehicle A crashed into vehicle B.

Better:
Vehicle A's front bumper lightly tapped vehicle B's rear bumper.

---

[12] *See e.g., State v. Amelio*, 197 N.J. 207, 214-15, 962 A.2d 498, 502 (2008). *See also State v. Guerrido*, 60 *N.J. Super.* 505, 511, 159 A.2d 448 (App.Div. 1960) ("[T]he average witness of ordinary intelligence, although lacking special skill, knowledge and experience but who has had the opportunity of observation, may testify whether a certain person was sober or intoxicated.").

[13] *See* Larry E. Holtz, *Promotional Exam Preparation Materials*, ESPOS: Educational Services for Preparing Officers and Supervisors (2018).

Report Writing in Special Cases 249

When describing a person with a disability, avoid using outdated, negative terms. New laws and regulations around the country have been replacing outdated and sometimes offensive pejorative terms with "person first" language, which, for example, refers to a person with a developmental disability" rather than a "developmentally disabled person." This is designed to emphasize a person's value, individuality, dignity and capabilities. It is therefore recommended that officials use terminology that maintains the respect and dignity of the person with special needs. The following guide has examples that will assist you in making the correct word choices.

TERMS NO LONGER USED	ACCEPTABLE TERMS
1. Handicapped person	1a. A person with a disability; or A person with special needs
2. The autistic kid	2a. A person with autism
3. The blind person	3a. A person who is blind
4. The disabled	4a. A person with a disability
5. Deaf and dumb	5a. A person who is deaf and cannot speak
6. Deaf-mute	6a. A person who is deaf and cannot speak
7. Deafness	7a. People who are deaf may have various issues: A person who is deaf but can speak. A person who is deaf and uses sign language. A person who is deaf and reads lips. A person who is deaf may also be called a person without hearing.

TERMS NO LONGER USED	ACCEPTABLE TERMS
8. Lunatic, insane, unsound mind incompetent; mentally defective; retarded; idiot; moron; half-witted; simpleton; imbecile	8a. A person who is mentally incapacitated; or A person with a cognitive disability. In some statutes, *"an incompetent"* is now described as a person who lacks the mental capacity to make a decision or waive rights.[14] The term *"mentally defective"* or *"insane"* has been replaced with *"a person with a mental disease or illness."*[15]
9. Mental defect	9a. In some statutes, this term has been replaced with: *A person who has "a mental disease or defect, which renders the victim temporarily or permanently incapable of understanding the nature of his conduct, including, but not limited to, being incapable of providing consent."*[16]

---

[14] In the laws related to Wills, Trusts and Estates, and Workers' Compensation, the terms "idiot," "lunatic," "mentally retarded," "feebleminded" or "insane" have been replaced with "a person who is mentally incapacitated."

[15] *See, e.g., N.J.S.*2C:13-4 (Interference with Custody).

[16] *See, e.g., N.J.S.*2C:12-10.2 (Stalking Restraining Order); *see also N.J.S.*2C:14-2a.(7) (Aggravated Sexual Assault).

Report Writing in Special Cases

TERMS NO LONGER USED	ACCEPTABLE TERMS
10. Bad speech Drunk-like speech Slurred speech; stroke speech Retarded speech Stutterer Computer speech	10a. A person with a speech impairment. **Note**: People with a speech impairment may also be referred to as: A person with a speech disability. A person with a communication disorder. A person with an assistive communication device.
11. Confined to a wheelchair Wheelchair bound	11a. A person who uses a wheelchair.
12. Cane guy	12a. A person who uses a cane.
13. Walker lady	13a. A person who uses a walker.
14. Cripple, crippled; spastic; spaz	14a. A person who has a physical disability; or A person who is physically disabled.
15. Deformed, freak or vegetable	15a. A person who has a physical disability; or A person who has multiple disabilities; or A person who has severe disabilities.
16. Nut-ball, insane, psycho, wacked, mental, deranged	16a. A person who has a mental illness; or A person with a behavior disorder; or A person with a personality disorder; or A person with a psychiatric disability.

TERMS NO LONGER USED	ACCEPTABLE TERMS
17. Mongoloid	17a. A person with Down Syndrome.
18. Epileptic, having fits	18a. A person with epilepsy; or A person with a seizure disorder.
19. Burn victim	19a. A person with a burn injury.
20. Birth defect	20a. A person with a congenital disability.
21. Deinstitutionalized	21a. A person who used to live in an institution.
22. Midget; gimp	22a. A person of short stature; or A little person; or A person with dwarfism; or A person who is a dwarf.
23. Alzy; demented; old-age disease	23a. A person who has dementia; or A person who has Alzheimer's disease.
24. A victim; sufferer; the stricken; sad; afflicted; troubled; an unfortunate; suffering from	24a. A person with an impairment or disability.

Knowing how to use appropriate terms to describe your interaction with a person with special needs, whether on the street, in a home or during an interview is essential. The following phrases may be used in reports that effectively describe how a special needs person interacted. Ask yourself these questions then use the information to help you write your report.

Report Writing in Special Cases 253

Why is this important? You need to determine if the person has the ability to process simple commands. It is important to determine if the individual has the ability to process and understand what is asked. If they have difficulty following your verbal directions it may indicate some type of disability. This would have significant impact on the person's ability to waive their *Miranda* rights and on their ability to provide a voluntary, knowing and intelligent consent to search. If they have difficulty processing information, or struggle with words and the flow of speech they may be an unreliable source of information. Recognizing these indicators provides you with essential information about the individual and their level of functioning. You are not required to diagnose or determine the person's disability. Just recognizing what they can and cannot do is important and relevant in your report. Strive to just report the facts. Ask the right questions and you have answers to the essential pieces of information. Even a negative response or incorrect response gives you important information.

Does the person speak?
(Always have a pad of paper and a pencil or pen available. If the person is deaf or unable to speak you can write out your questions and they can write their responses. This would be problematic if the person cannot read or write. Sometimes people with a physical disability are unable to speak, if they have a communication device allow them to use it.)

Did the person know their name?

Were they oriented to time and place?
This means did they know what time of day it was, what year, what season, what month?

Did they know where they were?

Do they know where they live?

Did they know who the president was?
An answer of "that guy," is the wrong answer.

Can they write their name?

Can they read a sentence?

Can they read something from a newspaper or book?

Do they have difficulty remembering the names of objects?

Can they identify simple objects?

Can they do a simple math problem?

Can they write the numbers asked?

Do they understand spoken language?
  Do they understand English?

Can they hear?

Do they appear confused?

Do they rock back and forth?

Do they fixate on an object and keep looking at it?

Do they appear limited in strength?

Are they alert?

Do they have coordination problems?

Do they repeat things over and over?

Do their hands shake?

Do they have other tremors?

Can they identify shapes?

Can they look at things as requested?

Do the responses to your questions make sense, are they relevant?

If you ask the person to name a fruit and the answer is a car, it indicates limitations. Put that in your report. Why? Because that simple response of "car" tells you they don't understand. Repeat the question, wait for another response. You can say, "I like bananas, Do you like any other fruits?" See how he or she responds; remember wrong answers tell you as much as correct responses. Always include this information in your report. Are the answers correct? Are they child-like? If the person appears to be in their thirties and the responses to your questions are those of a child, it tells you that the person's functional level is not that of an adult. A special-needs advocate may be needed for this individual.

§9.14. Keep It Short and Simple

The proper use of words also dictates that you should strive to avoid "double talk." If it's worth saying, it's worth saying once! Adding language that merely repeats what has already been said is a measure that detracts from the overall quality of the report.[17]

Examples of "Double Talk"[18] (Redundant Language)

advance warning	mix together
9:00 p.m. at night	final outcome
unexpected surprise	untrue lie
return again	return again
100% unanimous	so forth and so on
first time ever	month of July
over and done with	really truly
right beside	mutual cooperation
6:00 a.m. in the morning	stalling for time
each and every one	first start
usual custom	true fact
revert back	one and the same
separate out	rock back and forth
repeat over again	extra additions
rarely ever	end result
rise up	equally as important

---

[17] For more examples, *see* Larry E. Holtz, *Promotional Exam Preparation Materials*, ESPOS: Educational Services for Preparing Officers and Supervisors (2018).

[18] *Id.*

important essentials	other alternative
regular routine	few in number
most unique	blue in color
completely destroyed	sum total
may possibly	satisfactory enough
circulate around	square in shape
small in size	the reason is because
yelling and screaming	

Wordy vs. Concise [19]

Wordy	Concise
at that point in time	then
ahead of schedule	early
I am in possession of	I have
in advance of	before
made an escape	escaped
it is my opinion that	I think
all of a sudden	suddenly
until such time as	until
in the event that	if
provided that	if
on the condition that	if
at a later date	later
due to the fact that	because
the reason why is that	because
owing to the fact that	since
had occasion to be	was
take into consideration	consider
did not pay attention to	ignored
as a matter of fact	in fact
in spite of the fact that	although
there is no doubt but that	no doubt
first of all	first

---

[19] *Id.* at 65.

Report Writing in Special Cases

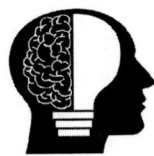

KEY POINTS

- When responding to incidents involving persons with special needs, one of the most important responsibilities of the first responder is report writing—the proper documentation of what was seen, heard and accomplished.

- For report writing, to maintain a proper frame of reference, the writer must not only assess an event from his or her perspective but must also determine how something may be perceived by others.

- Reports may be viewed by supervisors, the media, social service agencies, physicians, psychiatrists and insurance companies. In the criminal justice system, an officer's report will be read and analyzed by prosecutors, defense attorneys and judges.

- Report writing essentials include:
  - ~ Proper documentation
  - ~ Maintaining a proper frame of reference
  - ~ Ensure proper tone

- When responding to incidents involving persons with special needs, your field notes may serve as your first-responder's official memory. Whether taken in an actual notebook, iPad, audio recorder or similar device, field notes are a critical part of the process.

KEY POINTS (Continued)

- Reports should identify the:

    ~ "what and where"
    ~ circumstances
    ~ actions taken
    ~ resolution

- Reports describe an event that has a beginning, a middle, and an end.

- Be sure to include all relevant and necessary facts.

- Report writing should avoid legal and medical conclusions.

- Reports should contain appropriate words; outdated descriptions must not be used.

- Reports should use acceptable terms, and "person first" terminology.

- Use concise and precise words.

Chapter Ten
WHERE DO WE GO FROM HERE?

§10.1. No Encounter Is the Same

Interacting with the most vulnerable populations is never easy. Every day law enforcement officials, firefighters, EMTs, paramedics and first responders encounter persons with special needs. When responding to a call at a nursing home, an expectation of what you will encounter when you arrive is usually accurate. Arriving at a crime scene, an accident or other event does not give you a heads up on who and what you will encounter. Every one of us at some time in our lives will have a family member, a friend, a child, a coworker or a neighbor that has one or more of the special needs described in this book. Every one of us would hope that our special person be treated with fairness, respect and dignity. This book is an effort to help those important people who put their lives on the line every day, to serve and protect the citizens of this country when responding to incidents involving the unique needs of persons with special needs.

This book provides a history of special needs, and the laws that cover special needs. It identifies the impairments, explains the causes and provides essential information on response and assessment. The characteristics and behaviors of individuals with various types of special needs are detailed and guidelines for effective interactions are presented. The book is a resource tool, which can assist in training and education to improve the methods and interactions for responding to people with special needs. The suggestions, tips and methods are simply guidelines for positive interactions.

§10.2. The Legislative Initiative

Encountering an individual with disabilities or special needs in the field presents a challenge for any first responder. The media is quick to air events that have gone terribly wrong; and the images are played over and over by the media. In a world where there is 24/7 news coverage, an event that may have been buried in a newspaper in years past, is now a headline, sensationalized as news, and played repeatedly on YouTube.

This is one of the new realities facing all of us—the possibility that any encounter may be caught on video. Body cameras also record events as they happen. Someone is always looking over your shoulder. One's worth is measured in seconds and minutes. This is the new challenge facing today's law enforcement professionals, firefighters, paramedics, EMTs and other responders.

In an effort to minimize such negative circumstances with the disabled, the states of Alaska, New Jersey, Connecticut, Louisiana, South Carolina and Washington have enacted legislation or established policy, which now requires specific training to educate officers in encountering individuals with special needs. For example, Connecticut's Public Act No. 17-166 specifically addresses law enforcement training related to "juveniles with autism spectrum disorder or nonverbal learning disorder." Similarly, Louisiana's law, Act No. 210, requires training for "law enforcement interaction with persons with mental illness and persons with developmental disabilities." Although not a specific piece of legislation, New Jersey's Attorney General now requires all law enforcement officials to be trained in accordance with Law Enforcement Directive No. 2016-5, which now includes "Crisis Intervention Training and Responding to Persons with Special Needs."

Washington State has a particularly detailed legislative requirement in its Laws 2017, c. 295, (HB 1258). The new legislation is thorough and inclusive; it specifies training not only for fire department and emergency medical service personnel, but also for social and health services, state police patrol, sheriffs, police chiefs and the council of police and sheriffs. The new law is known and cited as the "Travis Alert Act," and according to its sponsor, Rep. Gina McCabe, it assesses the resources necessary to improve the Enhanced 911 program so that information pertaining to an individual's disability or special needs can be available to first responders before they arrive to the scene of an emergency. It would also require the Department of Health—in concert with other agencies—to review existing procedures and create a training program for first responders, providing instruction for how to best respond to emergencies involving persons with special needs. The act is named after Travis King, a 12-year-old boy with autism from Wapato, WA. This act is "the first step taken" in Washington state to "give first responders the critical tools and information they need to effectively help individuals with special needs in emergencies," said Rep. McCabe.

Alaska's House Bill No. 16, Chp.8, SLA 17 (§18.65.220) establishes detailed curriculum requirements for training police, probation, parole, and municipal correction officers. It specifies the importance of recognizing disabilities and appropriate interactions between police and the disabled. It is an excellent piece of legislation that recognizes and incorporates the critical elements to ensure the safety of this population.

As more states begin to adopt these practices and require such training, the challenge will be in creating a new set of policies, guidelines and procedures to address appropriate interactions between first responders and persons with special needs. An example of those components that may be included in effective public safety policy is set forth below. It may be utilized by those public safety officials looking to formulate new policy and training initiatives.

§10.3. Public Safety Policy

It is recommended that public safety agencies establish policy for agency personnel to properly respond to persons with special needs or persons who are disabled. To ensure the safety and well-being of such individuals, the policy must require appropriate and sufficient in-service training for a vast array of first responders and other public safety officials who may interact with such persons. Such training must include all police officers, sheriff's officers, probation and parole officers, bail officers, firefighters, EMTs, corrections officers, customs officials, court personnel, medical personnel and other first responders. In addition, this list should include the 47,000 Transportation Security Officers employed by the TSA.

Training modules for an appropriate response to incidents involving persons with special needs should, at a minimum, include:

- an explanation of disabilities, special needs and the terms used;

- instruction on disabilities that may include anyone with a medical, physical, emotional, behavioral, cognitive, developmental, sensory or speech disability;

- instruction on visible disabilities, or invisible disabilities and their accompanying special needs;

- guidelines on what to observe;

- guidelines on specific methods to de-escalate a situation;

- requirements of the American with Disabilities Act;

- resources available to persons with disabilities;

- techniques, protocols and best practices for interacting with persons who are disabled or have special needs;

- recognizing the need for medical or psychiatric intervention when required; and

- the option for communities to be able to minimize costs by sharing services, training and specialized personnel.

Accordingly, effective response and safety is achieved only through proper training and education. The men and women who are tasked with safeguarding the public must be provided with sufficient resources and the necessary tools for an appropriate response. Promoting the public welfare includes everyone: first responders, the municipalities they serve and the legislative bodies that oversee their responsibilities.

§10.4. Who Are the People in Your Neighborhood?

Knowing who the people are in your community is critical. However, law enforcement, firefighters and first responders need help. Knowing where the disabled and special needs individuals live is essential. In a crisis, this information could save time and the lives of these individuals as well as the responders. How can this information be obtained? A limited number of municipalities have begun to develop a voluntary "Special Needs Directory" to assist first responders in the event of an emergency. This is an excellent idea. The best plan is to have information available in a usable format *before* an emergency.[1]

Various states have used registries to identify and locate people with disabilities by asking them or their caregivers to voluntarily enter information into a registry such as *Smart911*, designed to identify individuals who may require special assistance during emergencies. *Smart911* is a secure, national database supported by fees paid by public agencies. The services are available to anyone, but is especially of value for individuals who *self-identify* as having special needs. Emergency response personnel use this information to make better decisions and improve response time, and municipalities can sign up for advanced services that enables them to know who lives in their community that might require additional assistance in the case of an emergency. Several Disability and Health programs around the country are now encouraging people with disabilities to sign-up for *Smart911* or similar registries.[2]

---

[1] New Jersey has established, by statute (N.J.S.40:15A-2), a "Yellow Dot Program," which is designed to provide emergency responders with critical health and emergency contact information about program participants so that emergency responders may aid program participants when those individuals are involved in motor vehicle emergencies or accidents and are unable to communicate. A **Yellow Dot Program window decal** on a motor vehicle involved in a motor vehicle accident or emergency shall serve as notice to an emergency responder assisting the vehicle that the driver or any passenger in the vehicle may be a participant in a Yellow Dot Program established pursuant to this act. If a motor vehicle is involved in a motor vehicle accident or emergency, and a Yellow Dot Program window decal is affixed to the vehicle, an emergency responder at the scene of such accident or emergency is authorized to search the glove compartment of the vehicle for a Yellow Dot Program envelope and health information card.

[2] https://www.smart911.com.

A model of a Special Needs Directory is outlined below. It should be effectively communicated and publicized as a voluntary effort to aide and assist all citizens having special needs in your community. People should be made aware of the importance of this project, and it should be given a memorable name, such as, *The Helping Hands Initiative* or the *We Care Project*. If the community is informed of the intent and scope of the project, participation is encouraged. The information could be entered onto an encrypted and secured computer program that could be accessed by law enforcement, firefighters and other first responders when answering an emergency call. This saves time and also provides important information as to who may be at the particular household and whether the responder should be prepared to provide assistance to a person with special needs.

When providing information about the directory the following sample press release may be used.

> *Our community is launching **"The We Care Project"** to serve our citizens with special needs. In an emergency, law enforcement and first responders need to know if anyone in your home needs assistance due to any type of disability, a medical issue, or whether a person is in a wheelchair, uses a walker or oxygen, or may have Alzheimer's or autism. Having this information in an emergency is vital, particularly when every second counts. Having this information beforehand can save your life or the life of a loved one. This information will be kept confidential and will be used only in an emergency. Your voluntary cooperation is appreciated.[3] To participate, visit our website at: https://www_____.*

---

[3] One such program may be found in New Jersey. It is called "NJ Register Ready." This is New Jersey's "Special Needs Registry for Disasters." It allows state residents with disabilities and functional needs and their families, friends, caregivers and associates an opportunity to provide information to emergency response agencies so emergency responders can better plan to serve them in a disaster or other emergency.
See https://www13.state.nj.us/SpecialNeeds/Signin?ReturnUrl=%2fSpecialNeeds%2f

Similarly, Rhode Island has created the Rhode Island Special Needs Emergency Registry (RISNER). This registry is designed to identify individuals who may require special assistance during emergencies, such as people with disabilities, long-term medical conditions, like diabetes, heart disease, and epilepsy, and other special healthcare needs. The information submitted to the RISNER is shared with local and state first responders and emergency management officials. The Department of Health and Rhode Island Emergency Management Agency have worked with E-911 to notify first responders when they are responding to a household that may have someone enrolled in the state registry.
See http://health.ri.gov/emergency/about/specialneedsregistry.

Model of Special Needs Directory

Name of Family
Address
Phone Number
Cell Number
Work number(s)
Email
Number of people in the home
Name and age of the person with the Special Needs
Disability (describe)
Characteristics and behaviors
Does the person use a wheelchair, walker, canes, crutches?
Does the person have a service animal?
Medical issues, symptoms, e.g., breathing problems, asthma, diabetic, etc.
Does the person need medication?
If so where can the medication be found?
Is the person fearful of uniforms?
Is the person fearful of emergency lights, sirens?
Can the person speak?
Does the person have a communication device?
Would the person hide in an emergency?
If they hide, where would they be likely to go? Specify which room or closet, etc.
If the person is not ambulatory or needs assistance with mobility, where would they most likely be located?
If the person needs oxygen where are the tanks located?
Is the person likely to run or wander?[4] Explain.

---

[4] Note that some states have established through legislation assistance in locating missing vulnerable persons. For example, in New Jersey, through P.L.2015, c.184, eff. 5-1-16, the legislature mandated that the Attorney General establish an "MVP Emergency Alert System," which will provide practices and protocols for the rapid dissemination of information regarding a person who is believed to be a missing vulnerable person. A "missing vulnerable person" or "MVP" is defined as a person who is believed to have a mental, intellectual, or developmental disability who goes missing under circumstances that indicate that the person may be in danger of death or serious bodily injury. The program would be a voluntary, cooperative effort between State and local law enforcement agencies and the media. *See* N.J.S. 52:17B-194.9; -194.10; -194.11

Please provide any other information you think is important (for example, our son has a favorite stuffed toy and doesn't feel safe without it).

Thank you for your participation in this life-saving project.

§10.5. An Ongoing Analysis

Determining whether an individual has a disability is a difficult task. Add to that difficulty is the fact that law enforcement officers out in the field many times need to make split-second decisions in tense, rapidly evolving situations. Keep in mind that an individual with a disability may act out or behave differently than others at the scene. Always, be alert to those differences.

The suggested methods, techniques and processes in this book may be used at any time to help a law enforcement officer, firefighter, paramedic, EMT and other first responders determine very rudimentary and basic functional capabilities of an individual with special needs. While they seem to be very simple, remember that the measurement of intellectual capacity and emotional intelligence is not an exact science. The methods are meant as a simple, quick guide to assist the officer in dealing with an individual with special needs. It is not a measurement device but a simple quick reference to provide helpful tips on what to do or not do when responding to incidents involving persons with special needs.

§10.6. An Ongoing Effort

In an effort to provide the support for the men and women who serve, serious consideration should be given by municipalities to share the services and costs in relation to special needs liaisons who may be available 24/7 by phone. These individuals would be available to all public safety officials, law enforcement, firefighters, paramedics, EMTs and other first responders. In certain circumstances, the best option would be to call for assistance. Having mental health experts available by phone would also provide assistance to the official who is dealing with a critical situation on the street. The communication and cooperation of a close working relationship between the various public departments and the special needs liaisons would create a supportive infrastructure, and would have a significant positive impact in responding to persons with special needs.

Developing an effective infrastructure to support and respond to persons with special needs requires multiple steps. Municipalities sharing services is an effective and cost-saving method of sharing the provision of training and education as well establishing partnerships with special needs and mental health liaisons. The development of public safety policy and legislative initiatives is another step in creating an infrastructure, along with the creation and implementation of a special needs directory to complete the process.

The development of a comprehensive training program, supported by an effective infrastructure of shared services, a database, as well as community and legislative support, may seem like a daunting task; but with any large project, it begins with first steps. As Stephen Covey aptly states in his book, *The 7 Habits of Highly Effective People*, "begin with the end in mind," that is, "start with a clear understanding of your destination. It means to know where you're going so that you better understand where you are now and so that the steps you take are always in the right direction."[5]

Now that we have a clear understanding of the specific elements and steps that are needed, each community may now develop its own methods and means of moving forward. Naturally, it will take time to put in place the necessary components. The process cannot happen overnight. What is important, however, is that you have already taken the first step.

---

[5] Stephen R. Covey, *The 7 Habits of Highly Effective People* (New York, NY : Free Press, 2004), p. 95, 98.

Glossary

Activities of Daily Living
A term used to describe a person's daily self-care activities. The term is used to describe a person's functional status in their ability or inability to carry out these functions. Examples of activities of Daily Living (ADL) are bathing, grooming, dressing, using the toilet, eating, drinking, and meal preparation.

Adaptive or Assistive Technology
Items that help people with a disability who have limitations such as speech, vision, hearing, or mobility.

Alzheimer's Disease
A type of dementia that causes problems with memory, thinking and behavior. The symptoms usually develop slowly and worsen with time. It is a progressive disease; in its early stages, memory loss is mild, but with late-stage Alzheimer's individuals lose their ability to carry on a conversation and respond to their environment. There is no current cure, but treatments for symptoms are available and research continues. Although current treatments can temporarily slow the worsening of the symptoms, they cannot stop the progression of the disease. The treatments can improve the quality of life for those with the disease. There is a worldwide effort underway to find better ways to treat the disease, delay its onset, and prevent it from developing. (alz.org)

American Sign Language
Sign language used by the deaf communities in the United States and most of Canada. American Sign Language (ASL) is a visual language. With signing, the brain processes linguistic information through the eyes. The shape, placement, and movement of the hands, as well as facial expressions and body movements, all play important parts in conveying information. (nad.org)

Americans with Disabilities Act of 1990
Provides a clear and comprehensive national mandate for the elimination of discrimination against individuals with disabilities. A more detailed explanation of the ADA may be found in Chapter Two.

Aphasia
An impairment affecting speech and language processing. It may also affect the comprehension of language and the ability to read or write. There may be difficulty with word retrieval, names of objects, word usage and flow of speech. It can be seen in children with brain damage and adults who have had a stroke. (aphasia.org)

Assistance Animals
The United States Department of Housing and Urban Development uses the term Assistance Animals in relation to the Fair Housing Act (FHA) as well as Section 504 of the Rehabilitation Act. It can include animals of various types that perform tasks or provide emotional support for individuals with disabilities.

Attention-Deficit/Hyperactivity Disorder (ADHD)
A brain disorder marked by an ongoing pattern of inattention and/or hyperactivity-impulsivity that interferes with functioning or development.

Auditory Processing Disorders
A learning disability characterized by difficulty understanding spoken language, processing what is heard, difficulty understanding and following verbal directions and is easily distracted by noise.

Autism
A "developmental disability significantly affecting verbal and nonverbal communication and social interaction, generally evident before age three, that adversely affects a child's educational performance. Other characteristics often associated with autism are engagement in repetitive activities and stereotyped movements, resistance to environmental change or

change in daily routines, and unusual responses to sensory experiences." 34 C.F.R. § 300.8(c)(1). Autism is a life-long disability. Also known as Autism Spectrum Disorder.

Cerebral Palsy
A neuromotor impairment, which damages the brain or nervous system. It is characterized by abnormal, involuntary and/or uncoordinated movements, which may or may not affect intellectual functioning. People with Cerebral Palsy may have difficulty speaking, require a wheelchair or other assistive device.

Child with a Disability
Refers to a child "having an intellectual disability, a hearing impairment (including deafness), a speech or language impairment, a visual impairment (including blindness), a serious emotional disturbance (referred to in this part as "emotional disturbance"), an orthopedic impairment, autism, traumatic brain injury, other health impairment, a specific learning disability, deaf-blindness, or multiple disabilities, and who, by reason thereof, needs special education and related services." 34 C.F.R. § 300.8(a).

Civil Rights of Institutionalized Persons Act (CRIPA) of 1980
The protection of the rights of people in state or local correctional facilities, nursing homes, mental health facilities and institutions for people with intellectual and developmental disabilities. Congress enacted this Act in 1980 to enable the Department of Justice (DOJ) to protect the rights of people residing in state institutions. The law authorizes the Attorney General to initiate or intervene in lawsuits in federal court to vindicate the rights of people in state-run or locally operated jails and prisons, juvenile correctional facilities, public nursing homes, mental health facilities, and institutions for people with intellectual disabilities.

Cochlear Implant
A cochlear implant is a small, complex electronic device that can help to provide a sense of sound to a person who is profoundly deaf or severely hard-of-hearing. The implant consists of an

external portion that sits behind the ear and a second portion that is surgically placed under the skin.

Cognitive Impairment
Cognitive impairment is any disorder that significantly impairs the cognitive function of an individual where typical functioning in society is difficult. Examples of some types of cognitive impairments: developmental disorders, motor skill disorders, amnesia, Alzheimer's Disease, substance-induced cognitive impairment, and some types of strokes.

Deaf-blindness – The complete inability to hear sound, complete inability to see.
Covers "concomitant hearing and visual impairments, the combination of which causes such severe communication and other developmental and educational needs that they cannot be accommodated in special education programs solely for children with deafness or children with blindness." 34 C.F.R. § 300.8(c)(2).

Deafness
A "hearing impairment that is so severe that the child is impaired in processing linguistic information through hearing, with or without amplification, that adversely affects a child's educational performance." 34 C.F.R. § 300.8(c)(3). Deafness is the complete inability to hear sound.

Degenerative diseases
A specific type of medical condition that causes tissues and organs of your body to change over time. Some degenerative diseases do not show up until later in life, such as Parkinson's and osteoarthritis, whereas muscular dystrophy affects children.

Deinstitutionalization
The name given to the policy through which the severely mentally ill, the severely cognitively impaired, and persons with multiple severe disabilities were moved out of large state institutions. As a result, many of the state facilities that served a real need closed. There was a belief that in doing this, patients could be served by their communities and that significant money could be saved in the process. Public psychiatric hospitals in

every state began to close. There were significantly less alternative facilities, community resources, and available placements for these populations. Some experts believe that the deinstitutionalization policy changed the mental health care system.

Dementia
A progressive disorder that effects the brain impairing a person's memory, ability to think and understand. It may cause communication problems, self-care abilities, mood, personality changes and behavioral issues.

Disability
Includes a "physical or mental impairment that substantially limits one or more of the major life activities of such individual"; a "record of such an impairment"; or "being regarded as having such an impairment." 29 C.F.R. §1630.2(g).

Disability Rights Education and Defense Fund (DREDF)
National law and policy center dedicated to protecting and advancing the civil rights of people with disabilities.

Dyscalculia
A learning disability characterized by difficulty with mathematics. grasping calculations, math processes and their applications.

Dysgraphia
A learning disability characterized by difficulty with handwriting and problems with holding a pencil, writing letters and word-spacing issues.

Dyspraxia
A developmental disability, which affects fine and or gross motor coordination. There may be issues with walking, balance, hand dexterity and speech.

Down Syndrome
Down syndrome (DS or DNS), also known as trisomy 21, is a genetic disorder caused by the presence of all or part of a third

copy of chromosome 21. It is typically associated with physical growth delays, characteristic facial features, and mild to moderate intellectual disability. This additional genetic material alters the course of development and causes the characteristics associated with Down syndrome. A few of the common physical traits of Down syndrome are low muscle tone, small stature, an upward slant to the eyes, and a single deep crease across the center of the palm—although each person with Down syndrome is a unique individual and may possess these characteristics to different degrees, or not at all.

Education for All Handicapped Children Act
Enacted by the United States Congress in 1975. This law had a transformative impact on millions of children with disabilities in each and every state in the country. The legislation required that public schools who received federal funds provide children with physical and mental disabilities a free and appropriate public education in the least restrictive environment.

Emotional Disturbance
A "condition exhibiting one or more of the following characteristics over a long period of time and to a marked degree that adversely affects a child's educational performance: (A) An inability to learn that cannot be explained by intellectual, sensory, or health factors; (B) An inability to build or maintain satisfactory interpersonal relationships with peers and teachers; (C) Inappropriate types of behavior or feelings under normal circumstances; (D) A general pervasive mood of unhappiness or depression; (E) A tendency to develop physical symptoms or fears associated with personal or school problems."

"Emotional disturbance includes schizophrenia. The term does not apply to children who are socially maladjusted, unless it is determined that they have an emotional disturbance." 34 C.F.R. § 300.8(c)(4). Emotional Disturbance can be life-long. Many adults with emotional disturbance have mental illness.

Emotional Intelligence
The ability to identify and manage your own emotions and the emotions of others. The skill requires the person to utilize emotion in problem solving and thinking.

Glossary

Emotional Support and Comfort Animals
These animals are not trained to perform specific disability-related tasks. They provide passive benefit; their presence is comforting to their owner.

Euphemisms
The substitution of an agreeable or inoffensive expression for one that may offend or suggest something unpleasant.

Every Student Succeeds Act 2015
Congress amended the Individuals with Disabilities Education Act (IDEA) through P.L. 114-95, renaming it the "Every Student Succeeds Act."19 In the law, Congress states: Disability is a natural part of the human experience and in no way diminishes the right of individuals to participate in or contribute to society. Improving educational results for children with disabilities is an essential element of our national policy of ensuring equality of opportunity, full participation, independent living, and economic self-sufficiency for individuals with disabilities. 20 U.S.C. §1415(f)(3)(C). Prior to the 2004 reauthorization, IDEA did not have a statute of limitations. *See Pub. L.* No. 108-446, 118 Stat. 2647.

Hearing Impairment
An "impairment in hearing, whether permanent or fluctuating, that adversely affects a child's educational performance but that is not included under the definition of deafness in this section." 34 *C.F.R.* § 300.8(c)(5). Hearing impairment is also seen in adults.

Impairment
A physical impairment is a physical disorder or condition, it could be a cosmetic disfigurement or anatomical loss affecting one or more of the body systems. A mental impairment is any mental or psychological disorder. A person could have an impairment from birth or it may be acquired. An impairment could be visible or not discernable.

Individual with a Disability
A person who has a physical or mental impairment that substantially limits one or more of the major life activities.

Individuals with Disabilities Education Act (IDEA) 1990

This Act was originally known as the Education of All Handicapped Children Act, which was passed in 1975. In 1990, amendments to the law were passed which changed the name to IDEA. In 1997 and again in 2004, additional amendments were passed to ensure equal access to education. The specifics of the law make available a free appropriate public education to eligible children with disabilities throughout the nation and ensures special education and related services to those children. The IDEA governs how states and public agencies provide early intervention, special education, and related services to more than 6.5 million eligible infants, toddlers, children, and youth with disabilities.

Infants and toddlers (birth through age two) with disabilities and their families receive early intervention services under IDEA Part C. Children and youth ages three through 21 receive special education and related services under IDEA Part B.

Reauthorization of IDEA. Under the IDEA, a plaintiff must file his or her request for an impartial due process hearing within two years of the date he or she became aware of the actions upon which her or his claims are based. The 2004 reauthorization of IDEA, which became effective July 1, 2005, amended the IDEA to include 20 U.S.C. §1415(f)(3)(C), which provides timelines for requesting hearings.

Intellectual Disability

A disability characterized by "significantly sub-average general intellectual functioning, existing concurrently with deficits in adaptive behavior and manifested during the developmental period, that adversely affects a child's educational performance. The term 'intellectual disability' was formerly termed 'mental retardation.'" 34 *C.F.R.* § 300.8(c)(6).

Intelligence Quotient IQ

A statistical score determined by standardized tests used to measure human intelligence.

Major Life Activities

Include, but not limited to: "(i) Caring for oneself, performing manual tasks, seeing, hearing, eating, sleeping, walking, standing, sitting, reaching, lifting, bending, speaking, breathing, learning, reading, concentrating, thinking, communicating, interacting with others, and working; and (ii) The operation of a major bodily function, including functions of the immune system, special sense organs and skin; normal cell growth; and digestive, genitourinary, bowel, bladder, neurological, brain, respiratory, circulatory, cardiovascular, endocrine, hemic, lymphatic, musculoskeletal, and reproductive functions. The operation of a major bodily function includes the operation of an individual organ within a body system." 29 C.F.R. §1630.2(i)

Mental Illness

Mental illness may affect emotional, psychological, and social well-being, thinking, mood and behavior. Some signs of mental health problems are: eating or sleeping too much, feeling numb, having low energy, feeling helpless, smoking, drinking or using drugs more than usual, feeling helpless or hopeless, mood swings, hearing voices, believing things that are not true, thinking of harming yourself or others, inability to perform daily tasks such as self-care. The Centers for Disease Control (CDC) reports that mental illnesses are among the most common health conditions in the United States.

One in five American adults experienced a mental health issue. One in 25 Americans live with a serious mental illness, such as schizophrenia, bipolar disorder, or major depression. Suicide is the tenth leading cause of death in the United States. It accounts for the loss of more than 41,000 American lives each year, more than double the number of lives lost to homicide. (mentalhelath.gov)

Miranda **Rights**

Prior to custodial interrogation, the person must be informed:
- You have the right to remain silent.
- Anything you say can and will be used against you in a court of law.
- You have the right to consult with an attorney and have an attorney present during questioning.
- If you cannot afford an attorney, one can be provided to you before questioning at no cost.

- You may ask for an attorney at any time during questioning, and questioning will stop if at any time you ask for an attorney.

Multiple Disabilities
Covers "concomitant impairments (such as an intellectual disability-blindness or an intellectual disability-orthopedic impairment), the combination of which causes such severe educational needs that they cannot be accommodated in special education programs solely for one of the impairments." The term "multiple disabilities" does not include deaf-blindness. 34 C.F.R. § 300.8(c)(7).

Muscular Dystrophy
A genetic condition that is hereditary, which leads to progressive muscle weakness and degeneration. As the disease progresses it becomes harder to move. It can be mild and progress slowly or severely and can be fatal. Presently, there is no cure, but different types of therapy and drug treatment can improve a person's quality of life and delay the progression of symptoms. (medicalnewstoday.com)

Musculoskeletal Disorders
Disorders that affect the movement of the human body's musculoskeletal system, which are muscles, tendons, ligaments, nerves, discs, blood vessels, etc. The disability can be from a limb amputation, fractures, joint or spine conditions, club foot, dwarfism, rheumatoid arthritis, paralysis, soft tissue injury (burns) as well as the many other specific conditions identified by the Social Security Administration.

No Child Left Behind Act of 2001 (NCLBA)
Designed to close the achievement gap with accountability, flexibility, and choice, so that no child is literally left behind. Through the NCLBA, Congress reauthorized the Elementary and Secondary Education Act; it included Title I provisions applying to disadvantaged students; and it supported standards-based education reform based on the premise that setting high standards and establishing measurable goals could improve individual outcomes in education.

Although the bill passed in the Congress with bipartisan support, it turned out to be such an unpopular law that, by 2015, the overwhelming criticism of the law caused Congress to strip away the national features of it. The NCLBA was replaced by the Every Student Succeeds Act and was turned over to the states to administer.

Orthopedic Impairment
A "severe orthopedic impairment that adversely affects a child's educational performance. The term includes impairments caused by a congenital anomaly, impairments caused by disease (e.g., poliomyelitis, bone tuberculosis), and impairments from other causes (e.g., cerebral palsy, amputations, and fractures or burns that cause contractures)." 34 C.F.R. § 300.8(c)(8).

Other Health Impairment
Having "limited strength, vitality, or alertness, including a heightened alertness to environmental stimuli, that results in limited alertness with respect to the educational environment, that: (i) Is due to chronic or acute health problems such as asthma, attention deficit disorder or attention deficit hyperactivity disorder, diabetes, epilepsy, a heart condition, hemophilia, lead poisoning, leukemia, nephritis, rheumatic fever, sickle cell anemia, and Tourette syndrome; and (ii) Adversely affects a child's educational performance." 34 C.F.R. § 300.8(c)(9).

Pejorative Terms
A word or phrase that has a negative connotation.

Personal Devices
Personal devices may include wheelchairs, prescription eyeglasses, hearing aids, computerized communication devices, braces, canes, and walkers.

Physical or Mental Impairment
Includes "(1) Any physiological disorder or condition, cosmetic disfigurement, or anatomical loss affecting one or more body systems, such as neurological, musculoskeletal, special sense organs, respiratory (including speech organs), cardiovascular, reproductive, digestive, genitourinary, immune, circulatory,

hemic, lymphatic, skin, and endocrine; or (2) Any mental or psychological disorder, such as an intellectual disability (formerly termed "mental retardation"), organic brain syndrome, emotional or mental illness, and specific learning disabilities." 29 C.F.R. §1630.2(g)

Reasonable Accommodation
(1) Covers: (i) Modifications or adjustments to a job application process that enable a qualified applicant with a disability to be considered for the position such qualified applicant desires; or (ii) Modifications or adjustments to the work environment, or to the manner or circumstances under which the position held or desired is customarily performed, that enable an individual with a disability who is qualified to perform the essential functions of that position; or (iii) Modifications or adjustments that enable a covered entity's employee with a disability to enjoy equal benefits and privileges of employment as are enjoyed by its other similarly situated employees without disabilities.

(2) Reasonable accommodation may include but is not limited to: (i) Making existing facilities used by employees readily accessible to and usable by individuals with disabilities; and (ii) Job restructuring; part-time or modified work schedules; reassignment to a vacant position; acquisition or modifications of equipment or devices; appropriate adjustment or modifications of examinations, training materials, or policies; the provision of qualified readers or interpreters; and other similar accommodations for individuals with disabilities. 29 C.F.R. §1630.2(o)

NOTE: A covered entity is required, absent undue hardship, to provide a reasonable accommodation to an otherwise qualified individual who meets the definition of disability. 29 C.F.R. §1630.2(o).

Rehabilitation Act of 1973, Section 504
The first disability civil rights law to be enacted in the United States. It prohibits discrimination against people with disabilities in programs that receive federal financial assistance and set the stage for enactment of the Americans with Disabilities Act.

Sensory Processing Disorder

A neurological disorder originally called Sensory Integration Dysfunction, whereby the brain has difficulty receiving and responding to information that comes from one or more of the five senses. It may cause sensitivity to loud sounds, bright or flashing lights, touch, texture and taste. May also cause hypersensitivity to the feel of some clothes, shoes, and the look, taste and or smell of food.

Service Animals

The ADA defines a service dog as one that is trained to perform "work or tasks" in the aid of a disabled person. A true service dog maintains the health and welfare of its human partner, and is considered a protected class under the Americans with Disabilities Act and Section 504 of the Rehabilitation Act. You must respond appropriately to someone using a service animal. Do not take the dog away. It is not considered a "pet." Do not touch the service animal when they are working.

Signed English

Sometimes referred to as Signed Exact English, a system of sign language used by a person who is deaf or hearing impaired. Signed English uses a sign for each word, so that the exact word of a spoken sentence is signed.

Silver Tsunami

The new term being used to describe the significantly increasing elderly population.

Social Intelligence

Develops from experience with people and learning from success and failures in social settings. It is more commonly referred to as "tact," "common sense" or "street smarts."

Special Education.

Includes specially designed instruction, at no cost to the parents, to meet the unique needs of a child with a disability, including (i) Instruction conducted in the classroom, in the home, in hospitals and institutions, and in other settings; and (ii) Instruction in physical education. May include: (i)

Speech-language pathology services, or any other related service, if the service is considered special education rather than a related service under State standards; (ii) Travel training; and (iii) Vocational education. 34 C.F.R. § 300.39(a).

Special Needs

One case has held that transportation companies and common carriers must render the necessary assistance to a person with special needs, such that "[w]here a passenger is blind, sick, aged, very young, [physically disabled], or infirm, and his condition is apparent or made known to the carrier, it is bound to render him the necessary assistance in boarding or alighting from its trains or cars." *McBride v. Atchison, Topeka & S.F. Ry. Co.*, 44 Cal. 2d 113, 119, 279 P.2d 966 (1955). A person with "special needs" is anyone who has an impaired ability to carry out the activities of daily living independently.

Specific Learning Disability

In general, a "specific learning disability means a disorder in one or more of the basic psychological processes involved in understanding or in using language, spoken or written, that may manifest itself in the imperfect ability to listen, think, speak, read, write, spell, or to do mathematical calculations, including conditions such as perceptual disabilities, brain injury, minimal brain dysfunction, dyslexia, and developmental aphasia." 34 C.F.R. § 300.8(c)(10). This definition "does not include learning problems that are primarily the result of visual, hearing, or motor disabilities, of an intellectual disability, of emotional disturbance, or of environmental, cultural, or economic disadvantage." *Id.*

Speech or Language Impairment

A "communication disorder, such as stuttering, impaired articulation, a language impairment, or a voice impairment, that adversely affects a child's educational performance." 34 C.F.R. § 300.8(c)(11). Speech impairments can be mild, moderate or severe, from mild articulation issues to the most severe, inability to speak.

Glossary

Spina Bifida

A neuromotor impairment that is a congenital birth defect in which the spinal column does not close all the way. The actual meaning of the words spina bifida means split-spine. As with other conditions, it can range from mild to severe to profound. Spina bifida can result in some paralysis. Intellectual functioning may or may not be affected. Some people with the condition may have difficulty walking, some may require a wheelchair and have problems with bowel or bladder control.

Standard Deviation

A standard deviation has been determined to be 15 points, which is possible on any IQ test. This means that a plus (+) or minus (-) of a 15-point variation is possible in either direction. When IQ tests were first developed, the mean was established at 100.

Stimming

Stimming is a shorthand expression for self-stimulatory behavior, which can be any type of repetitive movements of body parts, such as hand flapping, repetitive moving of objects or toys, repetition of words, phrases or sounds. It is a common characteristic in people with autism.

Substantial Limitation

A person who is unable to perform, or is significantly limited in the ability to perform, a major life activity that the average person in the general population can perform has a substantial limitation.

Supplemental Security Income Program (SSI)

SSI was established in 1972. It is a program that pays benefits to qualified disabled adults and children who have limited income and resources. It was signed into law on October 30, 1972, and went into effect in January 1974.

Therapy Animals

Therapy animals are trained by handlers and taken to various places such as hospitals, nursing homes, schools, and other places to provide therapeutic benefits for many people. We have seen them taken to places after a terrible tragedy to provide comfort to traumatized people. These animals are working animals but do not meet the ADA definition of a service animal because they do not serve one person with a disability.

Tourette's Syndrome
A neurological disorder characterized by repetitive, involuntary tics and vocalizations. Tics are often worse with anxiety or excitement.

Traumatic Brain Injury
An "acquired injury to the brain caused by an external physical force, resulting in total or partial functional disability or psychosocial impairment, or both, that adversely affects a child's educational performance. Traumatic brain injury applies to open or closed head injuries resulting in impairments in one or more areas, such as cognition; language; memory; attention; reasoning; abstract thinking; judgment; problem-solving; sensory, perceptual, and motor abilities; psychosocial behavior; physical functions; information processing; and speech. Traumatic brain injury does not apply to brain injuries that are congenital or degenerative, or to brain injuries induced by birth trauma." 34 C.F.R. § 300.8(c)(13).

Visual Impairment
An "impairment in vision that, even with correction, adversely affects a child's educational performance. The term includes both partial sight and blindness." 34 C.F.R. § 300.8(c)(13).

Visual Processing Disorder
Difficulty making sense of information seen through the eyes. The individual may have perfect vision; this is not a sight issue. It causes difficulty in the way the brain processes and interprets visual information. The eye may see a triangle, but the brain may interpret it as a square. Individuals may have a hard time recognizing the difference between objects, learning letters, numbers and learning to read.

References & Resources

References

10 Early Signs and Symptoms of Alzheimer's, reprinted with written permission from the Alzheimer's Association, https://alz.org/alzheimers-dementia/10_signs.

Alzheimer's and Dementia: What's the Difference? reviewed by Lisa Bernstein, MD., December 26, 2016. Retrieved June 4, 2018, from: WebMD Medical Reference, https://webmd.com.

Alzheimer's Facts and Figures Report, Alzheimer's Association, Retrieved June 4, 2018 from: https://www.alz.org/facts.

Americans with Disabilities Act of 1990, (ADA), Act of July 26, 1990, P.L. 101–336, 104 Stat. 327, which appears generally as 42 U.S.C. §§ 12101 et seq.

American Sign Language, The National Institute on Deafness and Other Communication Disorders (NIDCD) part of the National Institutes of Health (NIH), retrieved July 30, 2018, from: https://www.nidcd.nih.gov/American-Sign-Language.

Autism Data (2018, April 26) The Center for Disease Control and Prevention (CDC) Report, Retrieved June 11, 2018, from https://www.cdc.gov.ncbddd/autism/data.html.

Benet, William E, PhD., Psy.D. (2005, January) *Genius – An Overview,* retrieved July 30, 2018, from: https://www.assessmentpsychology.com/genius.htm.

Berman, Mark (2017, April 12) *Florida prosecutors charge police officer in shooting of autistic man's caretaker,* Retrieved June 11, 2018, from: https://www.chicagotribune.com/.../ct-charges-florida-officer-shooting-20170412-story.html.

Black, Edwin (2003, September) *The Horrifying American Roots of Nazi Eugenics,* Retrieved July 11, 2018, from: https://www.historynewsnetwork.org/article/1796.

Bouche Teryn, Rivard Laura (2014, September 18) *America's Hidden History: The Eugenics Movement,* Retrieved June 11, 2018, from: https://www.nature.com/.../america-s-hidden-history-the-eugenics-movement-12391944.

Bourne RRA, Flaxman SR, Braithwaite T, Cicinelli MV, Das A, Jonas JB, et al.; Vision Loss Expert Group (2017 September). *Magnitude, temporal trends, and projections of the global prevalence of blindness and distance and near vision impairment: a systematic review and meta-analysis.* Lancet Glob Health. 2017 Sep;5(9):e888–97.

Bureau of Justice Statistic Statistics, (2009 – 2015). *"Crime Against Persons with Disabilities, 2009 – 2015 Statistical Tables,"* NCJ 250632. Retrieved May 24, 2018, from https://www.bjs.gov/content/pub/pdf/capd0915st_sum.pdf.

Cannata, W. (2007) Autism 101 for Fire and Rescue, Retrieved June 11, 2018, from SPEAK Website, http://www.papremisealert.com.

Chuck, Elizabeth (2017, September 20) Associated Press, *"He Can't Hear You!": Deaf Man Shot Dead by Oklahoma City Police as Neighbors Scream in Horror*, Retrieved July 10, 2018, from: https://www.nbcnews.com/.../deaf-man-shot-dead-oklahoma-city-police-neighbors-scr...

Civil Rights of Institutionalized Persons Act of 1980 (CRIPA), Codified at 42 U.S.C. § 1997 et seq.

Classifications of Intellectual Disability Severity, as set forth by the National Library of Medicine. Retrieved July 26, 2018, from: https://www.ncbi.nlm.nih.gov/books/NBK332877/

Cochlear Implants, National Institute on Deafness and Other Communication Disorders (NIDCD), part of the National Institutes of Health (NIH), retrieved July 30, 2018, from: https://www.nidcd.nih.gov/health/cochlear-implants.

Crime Against Persons with Disabilities, 2009–2015 Statistical Tables, July 2017, Retrieved June 6, 2018, from: http://www.bjs.gov.

Crime Victims with Disabilities Awareness Act (P.L. 105–301).

Crisp, Quentin, "euphemisms quote," Retrieved May 25, 2018 from: https://www.quotes.net/quote/5003.

De Similien, Dr., Okorafor, Dr. (2017 May;16(5):47-52) Current Psychiatry, *Suicide by cop: What motivates those who choose this method?* Retrieved June 11, 2018, from: https://www.mdedge.com/psychiatry/article/136342/depression/...suicide-cop-what-motivates-those-who-choose-method.

Death of Eric Garner, Breathing Difficulty due to neck compression. (2014, July 17) Retrieved July 28, 2018, from:
https://www.en.wikipedia.org/wiki/Death_of_Eric-Garner

Dementia: Is this Dementia and what does it mean? Family Care Giver Alliance, Retrieved June 14, 2018 from: http://www.caregiver.org/fact-sheets.

Dementia, The Basics of Alzheimer's Disease and Dementia, U.S. Department of Health and Human Services, National Institute on Aging, Retrieved June 19, 2018, from: http://www.nia.nih.gov.

Deafness and Hearing Loss Fact Sheets, Retrieved June 18, 2018, from: https://www.who.int/news-room/fact-sheets/detail/deafness-and-hearing-loss. Also see: https:www.ada.gov/lawenfcomm.htm.,January 2006.

References & Resources

Disability Key Facts, World Health Organization, (WHO) Report of January 16, 2018. Retrieved July 11, 2018, from: http://who.int./news-room/fact-sheets/detail/disability-and-health.

Education of All Handicapped Children Act, P.L. 94-192; rev. P.L. 115-196. app. 7-7-18; *codified In Title 20 U.S.C. §1415*. Note that the Education of All Handicapped Children Act was *Later amended and renamed IDEA. See Pub. L. 101-476, §901(a), 104 Stat. 1141.*

Every Student Succeeds Act, *Pub. L. No. 114-95, 129 Stat. 1802, 2171 (2015).*

Federal Rule of Evidence 401.

Fentanyl Briefing Guide for First Responders, (2017, June) Retrieved June 11, 2018, from: https://www.dea.gov/.../Fentanyl_BriefingGuidefor First Responders_June2017.pdf.

Fishers Special Needs Directory, Fishers Fire Department, Fishers, Indiana https://www.fishers.in.us/219/Fishers-Fire_Department

Garner, Bruce (2017, November 17) *Training First Responders to Respond Better,* Retrieved June 7, 2018, from: https://www.eparent.com/features-3/training-first-responders-respond-bettter.

Grande, Laura.(2010, September 26) Strange and Bizarre: *The History of Freak Shows,* History Magazine, October/November Issue. Retrieved June 6, 2018, from: http://thingssaidanddone,wordpress.com/2010/9/26/stange-and-bizarre-the-history-of-freak-shows.

Gupta, Harsh (2016) *What Is The Highest IQ In The World Ever Recorded?* Retrieved July 30, 2018, from: https:www.scienceabc.com/ Also see http://sciabc.us/UTe7p.

Hartman, Steve (2014, May 23) As man's mind fades, heart comes to the rescue, Retrieved June 5, 2018, from: https://www.cbsnews.com/news/as-mans-mind-fades-heart-comes-to-the-rescue/

Hause, Melber (March 14, 2016) *"Half of People Killed by Police Have a Disability: Report,"* Retrieved May 24, 2018, from: https://www.nbcnews.com/.../half-people-killed-police-suffer-mental-disability-report.

Hause Marti, Melber, Ari, (2015, December 1) *Half of People Killed by Police Have a Disability: Report,* Retrieved June 11, 2018, from: https://www.nbcnews.com.../half-people-killed-police-suffer-mental-disability-report…quoting

Health & Education Statistics, National Institute of Mental Health, 2016, Bethesda, MD. Retrieved June 7, 2018, from: http://www.nimh.nih.gov/health/statistics/prevalence/any-disorder-among-children.shtml.

Helsel, Phil (2018, August 2) Police describe chaotic scene before veteran killed after self-defense shooting, Retrieved August 8, 2018, from: https;//www.nbcnews.com/.../police-describe-chaotic-scene-veteran-killed after-self-def...

Holtz, Larry E., *Interviews, Confessions and Miranda: Cases and Materials,* (Training Manual for Classes held in 2017 and 2018).

Holtz, Larry E., *Miranda in a Juvenile Setting: A Child's Right to Silence* (1987) 78 J. Crim. L. & Criminology 534, 536–537, 546–556.

Holtz, Larry E., (2018) *Promotional Exam Preparation Materials,* ESPOS: Educational Services for Preparing Officers and Supervisors.

How Common Are Specific Disabilities by Age?, United States Census Bureau Statistics, Retrieved June 6, 2018, from http://census.gov/programs-survey/acs/.

Hurst, Marianne (2005, May 17) *Handcuffing of Children Raises Questions, Unruly Elementary Pupils Pose Difficult Choices for Schools and Police,* Retrieved June 11, 2018, from: https://www.edweek.org/ew/articles/2005/05/18/37handcuffs.h24.html.

Illinois Premise Alert Program, Public Safety (430 ILCS 132/) PAP Act https://www.ilga.gov/legislation/ilcs.

Individuals with Disabilities Education Act, (IDEA), Codified at 20 U.S.C. § 1400 *et seq.* https://sites.ed.gov/IDEA/about-idea. See also https://www.sites.ed.gov/idea/regs/b/a/300.8/a.

Iverson, David M.D., Cornell, Marilyn MSW, Smits, Paul MSW, (2009, January 1) "The Army of Lost Souls" Retrieved May 24, 2018 from: https://journalofethics.ama-assn.org/article/army-lost-souls-commentary-1/2009-01.

Jin, Jill MD, MPH (2015, April 14) *Alzheimer's Disease,* The Journal of the American Medical Association, , retrieved June 29, 2018, from: https://jamanetwork.com/journals/jama/fullarticle/2247146.

The Journal of the American Medical Association, retrieved June 29, 2018, from: https://jamanetwork.com/journals/jama/fullarticle/2247146.

Journal of the American Medical Association: Family Care Giver Alliance, http://www.caregiver.org/fact-sheets.

Kelley, Erin, (2018, May 4). *The Sad Stories of the Ringling Brothers' "Freak Show" Acts,* pg.1., Retrieved on June 6, 2018 from: http://allthatisinteresting.com/freak-showmembers.

Kessler RC, Chiu WT, Demler O, Walters EE. Prevalence, *Severity, of Twelve-month DSM-IV Disorders in the National Comorbidity Survey Replication* (NCS-R) Archives of general psychiatry 2005;62(6):617-627.doi:10.1001/archpsyc.62.6.617. Substance Abuse and Mental Health Services Administration, Center for Behavioral Health Statistics and Quality (2016). Key substance use and mental health indicators in the United States: Results from the 2015 National Survey on Drug Use and Health, Rockville Maryland.

LaFave, Wayne R. (5th ed. 2012; 2017-2018 pocket part) *Search and Seizure: A Treatise on the Fourth Amendment* §8.2.

Lashley, Joel, (2013, March) Interventions for Patients with Challenging Behaviors, A Special Needs Subject Response for Police Officers, p. 4. Children's Hospital of Wisconsin, Security Services, Children's Hospital and Health Systems, Autism Spectrum Disorders: A Special Needs Subject Response for Police Officers. Form #95d2b2b5-41b9-40b5-951b-a5a3568696cc.

Learn about Mental Health, updated January 26, 2018, Retrieved June 16, 2018, from: http://www.cdc.gov/mentalhealh/index.htm.

Lester, D, (2015:4(1):1–6) Suicide as a Staged Performance, Comprehensive Psychology. Retrieved July 11, 2018, from: https://www.journals.sagepub.com

Mental Illness Policy Organization, *Law enforcement officers are the first responders to the Mentally Ill, and Suicide by Cop.* Retrieved July 10, 2018, from: https://mentalillnesspolicy.org/crimjust/law-enforcement-mental-illness.html.

Merriam Webster Dictionary, "euphemism" retrieved May 25, 2018 from https://www.merriam-webster.com/dictionary/euphemism.

Missing Vulnerable Person, "MVP Emergency Alert System" N.J.S.52:17B- 194.9; – 194.10; – 194.11.

Model Deaf Community, *"Do Deaf people consider themselves disabled?"* Retrieved May 25, 2018 from: https://www.modeldeafcommunity.org/?smart-faq=do-deaf-people-consider-themselves-disabled.

Morvay, Barbara J, (2010, February) *My Brother is Different: A parents' guide to help children cope with an Autistic sibling,* p. 4. (2010).

National Institute of Deafness and Other Communication Disorders (NIDCD), American Sign Language, Retrieved May 25, 2018, from: https://www.nidcd.nih.gov.

National Institute of Deafness and Other Communication Disorders (NIDCD), cochlear-implants, Retrieved May 25, 2018, from https://www.nidcd.nih.gov/health/cochlear-implants.

National Institute of Mental Health (NIMH), statistics on prevalence, treatment of mental illness in United States (January 1, 2018) Retrieved May 25, 2018, from https://www.nimh.nih.gov/health/statistics/index.shtml.

National Survey on Drug Use and Health (NSDUH) by the Substance Abuse and Mental Health Services Administration (SAMHSA), Data presented from 2016. Retrieved June 9, 2018, from: https://www.nimh.nih.gov/health/topics/index.shtml.

NBC News, *Florida Cop Charged with Manslaughter after Shooting,* Retrieved June 11, 2018, From: https://www.nbcnews.com...florida-cop-charged-manslaughter-shooting-autistic-man.

New Jersey Attorney General Directive No. 2015-1, *Regarding Police Body Worn Cameras (BWCs) and Stored BWC Recordings,* July 28, 2015 at p.3: http://www.nj.gov/lps/dcj/agguide/directives/2015-1_BWC.pdf.

New Jersey Register Ready, special needs registry for disasters, https://www.13.state.nj.us/SpecialNeeds/Signin.

N.J.S.2C:14-2a.(7). Aggravated Sexual Assault

N.J.S.2C:13-4. Interference with Custody

N.J.S.2C:12-10.2. Stalking Restraining Order

No Child Left Behind Act of 2001 (NCLBA), 115 Stat. 1425; codified in *Title 20* U.S.C. § 6842.

Nourse, Victoria, (2011). *Buck v. Bell: A Constitutional Tragedy from a Lost World,* 3 Pepp. L. Rev. 101–117.

Orthopedic Impairments, *Definition, Prevalence, Characteristics, Impact,* Retrieved July 26, 2018, from: http://www.projectidealonline.org/v/orthopedic-impairments/

Phillips, Noelle, (2018, July 13) The Denver Post, *Army Veteran Shot and Killed By Police After Defending Family from Naked Intruder.* Retrieved July 30, 2018, from: https://taskandpurpose.com/army-veteran-police-naked-intruder/

Ramos, Juan (2017, October 23) *Here is the Highest Possible IQ and the People Who Hold The World Record,* Retrieved July 12, 2018, from: https://www.sciencetrends.com/highest-possible-iq-people-hold-world-record/

Reilly, Ryan (2017, October 13) *Federal Judge Rules Handcuffing Little Kids Above the Elbows Is Unconstitutional,* Retrieved June 11, 2018, from: https://www.huffingtonpost.com/.../doj-handcuff-kids-kentucky_us_560ec5e5e4b076...

Reimann, Matt, (2017, June 15) Willowbrook, the institution that shocked a nation into Changing its laws, Patients needling "tenderness and affection" got the opposite, contributing writer. Retrieved June 6, 2018 from: http://Timeline_Now,timeline.com.

Rhode Island Special Needs Emergency Registry (RISNER) http://health.ri.gov/emergency/about/specialneedsregistry.

Rivera, Geraldo, (1972) *Willowbrook,* Retrieved June 6, 2018, Retrieved June 6, 2018 from: geraldo.com/folio/willowbrook.

Rui P, Hing E, Okeyode T, (2014). National Ambulatory Medical Care Survey: 2014 State and National Summary Tables. Atlanta, GA: National Center for Health Statistics, Centers for Disease Control and Prevention.

Ruben, Joel (2014, August 22) Pleading suspect dies in police custody: "You can breathe just fine" *Los Angeles Times.* Retrieved July 30, 2018, from: http://www.latimes.com/local/crime/la-me-lapd-custody-death-20140823-story.html.

Section 504 of the 1973 Rehabilitation Act, codified at 29 U.S.C. §794.

Service Animals, according to The ADA, retrieved June 27, 2018, from: https://www.ada.gov/regs2010/service_animal_qa.html. Also see the following http://www.adainfo.org/content/service-animals, Fall 2015.

Shortness of Breath, Trouble Breathing, known medically as dyspnea, (2018, January 18). *Causes, Basics and Symptoms,* Retrieved July 30, 2018, from: https://www.mayoclinic.org/symptoms/shortness-of-breath/basics/.../sym-20050890

Smart911, National database to identify and locate people with disabilities, requires registration and participation. https://www.smart911.com

Span, Paula (2017, July 24) *Another risk of aging: A police officer who doesn't recognize signs of dementia,* New York Times, Retrieved June 11, 2018 from: https://www.miamiherald.com/news/nation-world/national/article163372383.html

Specific Learning Disabilities categories and subcategories may be found at the government's. website: https://sites.ed.gov/idea/regs/b/a/300.8/a. The author's expanded detailed explanations are not part of the website.

Social Intelligence vs. Emotional Intelligence, (2017, October 13) i.e., XL, Exponential Learning Retrieved July 11, 2018 from: https://www.ie.edu/...social-intelligence-vs-emotional intelligence-making distinctions-...

Social Security Administration List of Adult and Childhood Impairments, for a comprehensive listing go to: https://www.ssa.gov/disability/professionals/bluebook/AdultListings.htm and https://www.ssa.gov/disability/professionals/bluebook/ChildhoodListings.htm.

Stern, Kenneth A., (2018, June 12) *Disability Etiquette,* Retrieved June 12, 2018 from http://www.cerebralpalsy.org/information/disability/etiquette.

Swanson, Jeffrey, PhD., McGinty, Elizabeth, PhD., Fazel, Seena, MBChB, MD., Mays, Vickie PhD. (2015, May). *Mental Illness and Reduction of Gun Violence and Suicide: Bringing Epidemiologic Research to Policy,* Retrieved June 7, 2018 from https://www.ncbi.nlm.nih.gov/pmc/articles/PMC4211925.

Swink, David F., (2010, October 2010) Communicating with People with Mental Illness: The Public's Guide, Retrieved July 11, 2018, from: https://www.psychologytoday.com/...management/.../communicating-people-mental-il...

The Greatest Showman, Chernin Entertainment (2017) https://www.bustle.com

Thirty-five Years of Progress in Educating Children with Disabilities Through IDEA, Archived: https://www2.ed.gov/about/offices/list/osers/idea35/history/index_pg10.html.

Torrey, Fuller, M.D., (posted 2005, May 10). "Deinstitutionalization: A Psychiatric Titanic," Retrieved May 24, 2018 from: https://www.pbs.org/wgbh/pages/frontline/shows/asylums/special/excerpt.html.

Traumatic Brain Injury, TBI, Definition and Symptoms, Retrieved July 26, 2018, from: https://medlineplus.gov/traumaticbraininjury.html.

Traumatic Brain Injury Characteristics, (2017, July 29) Retrieved July 26, 2018 from: https://www.mayoclinic.org/diseases-conditions/traumatic-brain-injury/symptoms-causes/

Treatment Advocacy Center (December 2015). *"Overlooked in the Undercounted, The Role of Mental Illness in Fatal Law Enforcement Encounters,"* p.1. Retrieved May 24, 2018 from: http://www.treatmentadvocacycenter.org/storage/documents/overlooked-in-the-undercounted.pdf

Tuohy, John (2017, April 17) *Registry will help Fishers firefighters rescue special needs victims,* Retrieved June 11, 2018, from: https://www.indystar.com+sory+registry+help+fisher+firefighters+rescue+special+needs.

Twain, Mark (Samuel Clemens) (1888, October 15) Letter to George Bainton, Retrieved June 1, 2018, from, https://www.twainquotes.com.

Vespa, Jonathan, (2018, March) U.S. Census Bureau, Population Projections, Retrieved June 11, 2018, from: https://www.census.gov/newsroom/press.../cb18-41-population-projections.html

What Causes Alzheimer's Disease? U.S. Department of Human Services, content reviewed May 22, 2017. Retrieved June 19, 2018, from: https://www.nia.nih.gov/health/what-causes-alzheimer's-disease.

References & Resources

What is Mental Illness? American Psychiatric, physician reviewed by Ranna Parekh, MD., M.P.H. (2015, November) Retrieved June 19, 2018, from: http://www.psychiatry.org/patients-families.

Willowbrook, *Unforgotten: Twenty-five Years After Willowbrook,* Retrieved June 6, 2018 from: http://www.youtube.com/watch/Unforgotten:Twenty-five Years After Willowbrook.

World Health Organization, (2018, January 16) *"Key Facts"* Retrieved May 24, 2018 from: http://who.int./news-room/fact-sheets/detail/disability-and-health.

Yellow Dot Program, established in New Jersey by statute (N.J.S.40:15A-2) Registry for emergency responders to assist disabled.

Resources

Alzheimer's Disease / Dementia

Alzheimer's Association
  www.alz.org

Alzheimer's Association's Safe Return Program?
  www.alz.org/caregiver/programs/safereturn.htm

Alzheimer's and Dementia Resources
  https:www.alzheimers.net/resources

National Institute on Aging NIA Alzheimer's and related Dementias Education and Referral (ADEAR) Center
  adear@nia.nih.gov
  www.nia.nih.gov/alzheimers.org

National Alzheimer's and Dementia Resource Center (NDRC)
  https://nadrc.acl.gov

Relieving Stress & Anxiety: Resources for Alzheimer's Caregivers
  https://www.nia.nih.gov/health/relieving-stress-anxiety-resources-alzheimers-caregivers

Alzheimer's & Dementia Resource Center
  https://adrccares.org/

Autism

Autism Speaks Organization
  www.autismspeaks.org/family-services/resource

Autism Research Institute
  www.autism.com

Autism Society of America
  www.autism-society.org

American Autism Association
  https://www.myautism.org

National Autism Center
  www.nationalautismassociation.org

Asperger Syndrome & High Function Autism Association
  ahany.org

References & Resources

Blindness or Visual Impairment

American Council of the Blind
www.acb.org

American Foundation for the Blind
www.afb.org

National Eye Institute
https://nei.nih.gov/lowvision/content/resources2

Deafness or Hard of Hearing

National Association of the Deaf
www.nad

National Institute on Deafness and Other Communication Disorders
www.nidcd.nih.gov

Alexander Graham Bell Association for the Deaf and Hard of Hearing
www.agbell.org

Disabilities

Americans with Disabilities Act Information Line
www.usdoj.gov/crt/ada/adahom1.htm

American Association on Intellectual and Developmental Disabilities
http://www.aaidd.org

Support for children with multiple disabilities
www.ncbi.nlm.nih.gov

Programs for People with Disabilities
www.hhs.gov/programs/social-services/...people-with-disabilities/index.html

Resources for People with Disabilities
www.benefits.gov

The Arc, for People with Intellectual and Developmental Disabilities
www.thearc.org

Easter Seals

Offers help and answers for children and adults living with autism, other disabilities and or special needs. Centers may be found throughout the United States.

www.easter-seals.org

United Cerebral Palsy
www.ucp.org

Disabled Peoples' International
www.dpi.org

March of Dimes Birth Defects Foundation
www.@macrchofdimes.com
www.marchofdimes.com

Social Security Administration
www.ssa.gov

Spina Bifida Association of America
www.sbaa.org

National Council on Disabilities
www.ncd.gov

National Rehabilitation Information Center (NARIC)
www.naric.com

Disability Rights Education & Defense Fund
www.dredf.org

US Equal Employment Opportunity Commission
www.eeoc.gov

Learning Disabilities

Learning Disabilities Association of America
www.ldaamerica.org

National Center for Learning Disabilities
www.ncld.org

National Institute of Health/Learning Disabilities Information Page
www.ninds.nih.gov/Disorders/All.../Learning-Disabilities-Information-Page

Firefighters

Special Needs Fire Prevention and Response Awareness - Firefighter ...
https://www.fireengineering.com/.../special-needs-fire-prevention-and-response-

Fire safety outreach materials for people with disabilities
https://www.usfa.fema.gov/prevention/outreach/disabilities.html

Medical Terms and Dictionary

https://medical-dictionary.thefreedictionary.com
https://dictionary.webmd.com
https://www.online-medical-dictionary.org

References & Resources

Mental Health and Mental Illness

National Institute of Mental Health
  www.nimh.nih.gov

NAMI - National Alliance on Mental Illness
  www.nami.org

Mental Health Information
  www.mentalhealth.gov

Mental Health America
  www.mentalhealthamerica.net

Mental Health Resources - Public Health
  https://www.publichealth.org/resources/mental-health

Neurological Issues

National Institute of Neurological Disorders and Stroke (NINDS)
  braininfo@ninds.nih.gov
  www.ninds.nih.gov

Social Security Administration Disability Determination Process
  https://www.ssa.gov/disability/determination.htm

Special Needs Registry

In addition to the National database for first responders found at Smart911.com, some cities and states have taken the initiative to create a special needs registry. Here are just a few:

Albany, New York, Functional Needs 911 Registry
  www.albanycounty.com

City of Fishers Special Needs Registry for First Responders
  www.fishers.in.us/219/Fishers-Fire-Department

Florida Special Needs Registry
  https://snr.floridadisaster.org/

New Jersey Special Needs Registry
  https://www13.state.nj.us/SpecialNeeds

Rhode Island Special Needs Emergency Registry: Department of Health
  www.health.ri.gov/emergency/about/specialneedsregistry/

Tarrant County, Texas, Special Needs Assistance Program (SNAP)
  www.accesstarrantcounty.com

Index

10 Early Signs and Symptoms of Alzheimer's Disease 44
Affirmative Dilemma. 201
ALS 64
Alzheimer's Association Safe Return® program 100
Alzheimer's Disease 44
   10 early signs and symptoms 48
American Civil Liberties Union 86
Americans with Disabilities Act 112
Americans with Disabilities Act of 1990 21
Aphasia 39, 156
Argyrophilic grain disease 43
Assistance animals 110
Auditory processing disorders 39, 156
Autism Spectrum Disorder 78
Autism Spectrum Disorder (ASD) 29
Bellis v. United States 180
Bertelsman, Judge William 92
Big Bang Theory 135
Blind and visually impaired 105
Bobby v. Dixon 186
Body-worn cameras 238
Bram v. United States 185
Breathing issues 160
Brewer v. Williams 175
Buck v. Bell 57, 130
Center for Disease Control and Prevention (CDC) 78
Centers for Disease Control (CDC) 48
Cerebral Palsy 148
Chronic traumatic encephalopathy (CTE) 43
Civil Rights of Institutionalized Persons Act (CRIPA) 20
Clewis v. Texas 187
Cochlear implant 33
Colorado v. Connelly 204
Consent
   co-occupants 218
   common authority 217
   express or implied 217
   obtaining 220-226
   scope 219
   voluntary or coerced 214
Consent to search 211
Cooper v. Griffin 197
Covey, Stephen 267
Creutzfeldt-Jakob disease 43
Crime Against Persons with Disabilities 74

Index

Crime Victims with Disabilities Awareness Act 73
Crisis Response Team 125
Custody 172
Darwin v. Connecticut 187
Davis v. United States 182
Deaf-Blindness 31
Deafness 31
Deafness and hearing impairment 111
Degenerative diseases 149
Deity Dilemma 205
Dementia 41
Diagnostic and Statistical Manual of Mental Disorders V, (DSM-5) 50
Dickerson v. United States 169
Disability Etiquette 65
Disability terminology 67
Drug epidemic 76
Due process 204
Dyscalculia 39, 157
Dysgraphia 40, 157
Dyslexia 40, 157
Dyspraxia 40, 157
Edison, Thomas Alva 132
Edwards v. Arizona 180, 182
Emotional disturbance 36
Emotional intelligence 131
Emotional support and comfort animals 109
Eugenics movement 129
Euphemisms 27
Every Student Succeeds Act 22
Fairmount Park Elementary School 93
Fentanyl 77
Florida v. Jimeno 219
Frazier v. Cupp 186
Freak shows 58
Gallegos v. Colorado 187
Garner v. Mitchell 194
General Tom Thumb 60
Georgia v. Randolph 218
Government's Individuals with Disabilities Education Act 28
Hawking, Stephen 64
Hearing impairment 36
HIV-associated dementia (HAD) 43
Huntington's disease 43
Illinois v. Rodriguez 226
Individuals with Disabilities Education Act (IDEA) 20, 22
Ingalls, Clyde 59
Intellectual disability 37, 129
Intelligence Quotient 130
Interrogation 173

Index 301

J.D.B. v. North Carolina 172
Learning disabilities; specific 155
Legislative initiative 259
Lou Gehrig's disease 65
Marshall, Randall 94
Maryland v. Shatzer 182
McBride v. Atchison, Topeka & S.F. Ry. Co. 282
McNeil v. Wisconsin 167
Medic alert 100
Mensa International 133
Mental illness 48, 121, 122
Michigan v. Mosley 179
Miller v. State 192
Miranda Rights 168
    custody 172
    formula 170
Miranda v. Arizona 168
Multiple disabilities 142
Multiple disability 37
Musculoskeletal disorders 149
Negative descriptive phrases 62
Negativity 68
Neurodegenerative disorders 42
Neuromotor impairment 148
New York v. Quarles 178
No Child Left Behind Act of 2001 (NCLBA) 21
Oregon v. Mathiason 173
Orthopedic impairment 37, 148
Other health impaired 38
Paraplegia 148
Pejorative terms 62
People v. Schoenhofen 193
Person with special needs 71
Political correctness 27
Progressive brain disease 42
Public safety policy 261
Reauthorization of IDEA 22
Report writing 231
    body-worn cameras 238
    checklist 240
    documentation 232
    field notes 237
    frame of reference 232
    include all facts 241
    inferences 245
    objective v. subjective 246
    proper tone 234
    short and simple 255
    shorthand expressions 244

Index

Rhode Island v. Innis 174
Right to refuse consent 213
Ringling Brothers' Circus 59
Rivera, Geraldo 61
Sensory processing disorder 40, 158
Service animals 108
    terminology 109
Sideshows 59
Sign language 34
Silver Tsunami 95
Smart911 263
Smith v. Illinois 181
Smith v. Mullin 195
Social intelligence 131
Special Needs Directory 264
    model of 265
Specific learning disability 38, 155
    subcategories 39, 156
Spina Bifida 149
State v. Flower 202
State v. Galloway 186
State v. W.S.B. 242
Stern, Kenneth A. 65
Stern, Ludwig Wilhelm 131
Suicide 121
Suicide by cop 124
Terman, Lewis Madison 131
Therapy animals 110
Traumatic brain injury (TBI) 158
United States v. Garibay 197
United States v. Grap 223
United States v. Richards 220, 232
United States v. Strache 226
United States v. Turner 196
Vespa, Jonathan 95
Visual processing disorder 40, 158
Voluntariness 184
Waiver of rights 183
We Care Project 264
Willowbrook School 60
World Health Organization 105
Youth Rights Form 188